Advance praise for *Personalized Exposure Therapy*

"*Personalized Exposure Therapy: A Person-Centered Transdiagnostic Approach* by Jasper Smits, Mark Powers, and Michael Otto, shares the secrets that every successful exposure therapist knows. The authors, rock stars of exposure therapy, explain the principles clearly, offer explicit guidelines to put them into action, and present clinical examples to bring these principles to life. This volume covers everything from assessment through treatment to termination, including suggestions of assessment instruments. It is very engaging, practical, and well written and details real life situations such as when medications are involved in exposure therapy. Every clinician who treats a patient with anxiety should read this cover to cover, and it will help them provide better treatment for the rest of their therapeutic lives."

—**Barbara O. Rothbaum, PhD, ABPP**, Professor in Psychiatry, Director, Veterans Program and Trauma and Anxiety Recovery Program, Paul A. Janssen Chair in Neuropsychopharmacology, Associate Vice Chair of Clinical Research, Emory University School of Medicine

"*Personalized Exposure Therapy* belongs in the hands of every clinician who wants to treat fear-based disorders successfully. In clear language, Smits, Powers, and Otto bring the principles of exposure therapy to life, with compelling case examples and a clearly articulated rationale. Clinicians of all levels will find a wealth of useful, practical information in this book."

—**David F. Tolin, PhD**, Director, Anxiety Disorders Center, The Institute of Living, and author of *Doing CBT: A Comprehensive Guide to Working with Behaviors, Thoughts, and Emotions*

"This book describes cutting-edge advances in cognitive science and integrates them with what is known from intensive clinical study to help clinicians design and provide the kind of treatment patients with anxiety disorders most need. At every step, the conceptual understanding is grounded in the examples, scripts, and handouts that make this book 'session ready' for clinicians and their patients. Unlike some manuals, this book is not a session-by-session treatment manual. Instead, it provides a comprehensive perspective on the principles and procedures behind exposure interventions."

—**Edna B. Foa, PhD**, Professor in Psychiatry and Director of the Center for the Treatment and Study of Anxiety, University of Pennsylvania Perelman School of Medicine

Personalized Exposure Therapy

A Person-Centered Transdiagnostic Approach

JASPER A. J. SMITS
MARK B. POWERS
MICHAEL W. OTTO

OXFORD
UNIVERSITY PRESS

OXFORD
UNIVERSITY PRESS

Oxford University Press is a department of the University of Oxford. It furthers the University's objective of excellence in research, scholarship, and education by publishing worldwide. Oxford is a registered trade mark of Oxford University Press in the UK and certain other countries.

Published in the United States of America by Oxford University Press
198 Madison Avenue, New York, NY 10016, United States of America.

CIP data is on file at the Library of Congress
ISBN 978-0-19-060245-1

JAJS: To Stella Smits, I love you and your attitude, "Live in the moment, not in the past or the future."

MBP: To my wife Kristin and her mantra, "Go to your fears and weaknesses for there your genius lies."

MWO: To Summer Ladd Otto and Samuel West Otto, I adore your brilliant and sensitive hearts.

Contents

Figures

Tables

Boxes

Personalized Exposure Therapy

1

Introduction

Making a Case for Personalized Exposure Therapy

1.1. What Is Exposure Therapy?

The beauty of exposure therapy is that it is anchored in theory, simple in principle, but rich in clinical innovation. And it works. Most clinicians would agree that it makes sense to reintroduce a patient to avoided and feared cues when the goal is to help that individual rid himself or herself of anxieties and return to a fulfilling life. The goal is to create a renewed sense of safety around once-feared cues, helping the patient recognize that harm is unlikely and be willing to take minor "risks" because doing so yields a life that is more rewarding.

Some sort of exposure is always part of successful treatment of anxiety and related disorders, because patients eventually need to re-enter avoided situations to return to full engagement in life. As compared to naturalistic exposure, exposure therapy is a well-designed procedure for maximizing the therapeutic learning of safety that comes from successful exposure. In exposure therapy, patients learn anew the safety of situations and events, as well as their own ability to cope and thrive in these situations. There are a variety of ways of learning safety. Some clinicians prefer a cognitive approach that relies on the careful evaluation of thoughts. Yet, even richly cognitive approaches are not conducted in a vacuum; they are instead conducted in the context of active monitoring of ongoing experience.

This experience is exactly what is provided by exposure therapy. Exposure is programmed experience, plain and simple—guided experiences to help individuals undo the faulty, maladaptive, and anxiogenic beliefs; vigilance to harm; and avoidance that characterize anxiety and related disorders. Exposure therapy is an especially malleable approach and can provide a "where the rubber meets the road" addition to almost any therapy. That is, regardless of whether clinicians see themselves as leading therapy with an eclectic, supportive, humanistic, or cognitive therapy approach, as long as the clinician is willing to facilitate active learning episodes, exposure therapy can be integrated within treatment and can speed a therapeutic response.

For such a straightforward concept, exposure therapy has garnered a wide range of misconceptions in its years of use. To clarify our understanding of exposure therapy, we review what we believe are the top five misconceptions about exposure interventions. In no particular order, these misconceptions include:

(1) *Exposure is a brain-dead process that relies on simple repetition and that makes little use of my patients' abilities as engaged and thinking individuals.* Research over the last two decades has made it clear that exposure-based learning (fear extinction) does not involve the successive weakening of fear associations; instead it is an active process of learning safety in response to fear cues. As an active learning process, full engagement of a range of strategies for creating and setting-in memories of safety is important. Safety learning, like other learning processes in humans, engages both automatic (unconscious) and strategic (conscious) cognitive processes, and results in learning outcomes that rely on both automatic and effortful behavioral outcomes.

In this book, we pay attention to safety learning that occurs as part of both of these—automatic and strategic—processes. Indeed, Chapter 2 is entitled "Thinking through Exposure" not just because it provides a conceptual overview to clinicians on how to think about exposure, but because it guides clinicians on how to help their patients *think* actively before, during, and after the exposure exercises. The exposure session provides a core opportunity for safety learning in the context of ongoing experience, but this learning is enhanced by active engagement of cognitive resources to help consolidate and extend these gains.

(2) *Exposure is a one-size-fits-all procedure that may not be appropriate for my particular patients.* It is true that exposure relies on a one-size-fits-all *core principle*, because the principle of fear extinction has been validated repeatedly across not only thousands of individuals but across multiple species. However, it is not true that the exposure interventions (used to engender fear extinction) are unitary across patients. Part of the thrust of this book is to show the importance of tailoring the exposure exercise to an individual's core fears and the particular contexts that modulate these fears (i.e., case formulation). Quite easily, a clinician may never do exposure practice the same way twice, given how important it is to fit the exposure exercises to the specific safety learning needed by a particular patient. In addition, surveys of clinicians have revealed deep misgivings about treatment manuals, with complaints such as "manuals may not be appropriate for the complex and unique patients in a particular clinical practice," "a fixed 16-session approach is too rigid," "a fixed approach is difficult to incorporate into ongoing treatment with a patient," "manuals don't give guidance on what to do if the session unfolds differently

than what is depicted in the manual," or "manuals stifle creativity and innovation."

In response to concerns like these, we have not written a treatment manual. We have instead written a principle- and procedure-based guide for the delivery of exposure therapy that encourages exposure planning around the unique fear characteristics of an individual patient. Our book is not organized around diagnoses, instead, it is organized around (a) the case formulation that leads to the identification of a specific set of fears, concerns, behaviors, and contexts that will be the target of safety learning and (b) the development of exposure experiences that are guided by principles and examples but are unique to each patient. These exposure interventions can be added on to any program of ongoing treatment. As such, this book is designed to help clinicians bring state-of-the-art exposure interventions to whatever stage of therapy a clinician may find himself or herself with a patient.

(3) *Exposure is too hard on patients; don't a lot of patients drop out of exposure treatment?* Ongoing study shows that exposure therapy is an especially tolerable treatment, with strong retention of patients in treatment relative to both medication alternatives as well as the attrition rates observed in open-treatment care networks. We believe this occurs because exposure-based treatments start with a clear rationale, provide incremental treatment benefits, and can be readily modified should patients face barriers to progress. Moreover, when clinicians ask for an initial investment of a fixed number of sessions and engage patients in the active monitoring of treatment outcome, treatment benefits are especially palpable relative to a patient's investment in therapy. Indeed, examination of session-by-session outcomes shows that initial benefit is realized by many patients in the very first session, with continued benefit thereafter. In addition, in exposure therapy, some patients experience sudden gains (when they achieve over 50% improvement across a single week of treatment) that are driven by a reconceptualization of their fears and their resilience following a single exposure session. Accordingly, both incremental and sudden gains provide patients with anxiety relief, a return to more functional activity, and motivation to continue with the methods that work. Each of these gains provide motivation for continued work with exposure therapy.

(4) *Exposure therapy is so challenging, patients need to be on medication first.* This misconception about exposure therapy should be considered in relation to its psychosocial analogue, "When a person feels anxious, doesn't this mean that he or she needs more coping responses?" We will consider both forms of these concerns together, because they share the same root concern—that the patient needs to be protected from his or

her own experience of anxiety. We agree that being afraid of one's own emotional responses is an especially debilitating and overwhelming condition, and this condition needs good treatment. This treatment, we believe, is not to engage the patient in additional avoidance of his or her own emotional experience, but to intervene to reduce the aversiveness of his or her experience of anxiety as a first step toward decreasing the frequency and intensity of anxiety. Chapter 5 emphasizes the transformation in the personal meaning of anxiety that comes from exposure interventions targeted specifically to the experience of anxiety/panic itself (interoceptive exposure). This approach ensures that coping responses are learned in relation to making anxiety more tolerable, while patients are learning safety. Furthermore, it is the role of personalized treatment planning to ensure that any of the "steps" in safety learning to feared cues are not so large that the patient feels exposure practice is not possible. Exposure practice always starts where the patient is and steps forward in a reasonable way from that point. It is true that anxiety medication may be chosen by some patients to aid their entry into therapy, but this represents a personal preference rather than a desirable treatment strategy for the following reasons: (a) there is not supportive evidence that the addition of medication to exposure improves treatment adherence, perhaps due to the complicating factors of medication side effects; (b) considering the "need" for medication to ease the process of exposure, there is evidence that treatment with antidepressants and benzodiazepines, while offering benefits on their own, may in fact slow treatment benefit from exposure-based treatment and add substantially to the costs of treatment; (c) the addition of medications to exposure-based treatment also appears to detract from the staying power of the exposure; when medications are later discontinued, the risk of relapse is dramatically higher unless the exposure-treatment is reinstated before, during, and after the medication taper period. Indeed, medication combination issues are so complex that we devoted Chapter 8 to elucidating strategies to best manage combination treatment strategies.

(5) *If a patient has failed to get better with exposure on his or her own (or with a past clinician), doesn't that mean that exposure won't work and other interventions should be offered?* It is true that many patients will have persisted for years, working to enter feared situations prior to finally coming to therapy. Indeed, in one of our studies, we documented that patients had struggled with their disorders for over a decade before coming to our treatment. These patients got better rapidly, raising the question about why their own persistence in the face of anxiety did not lead to a cure. The answer lies in how you approach exposure. Effective

exposure is not a process of "grinning and bearing it" or of "cheating one's way through a hard situation." It is a process of evaluating what happens when subtle avoidance behaviors are eliminated in favor of testing how safe the situation truly is. These subtle avoidance behaviors are termed "safety behaviors" because they create a *false* sense of preventing feared outcomes, and thereby *prevent a fuller learning of real safety in feared situations*. Elimination of safety behaviors and a focus on objective evaluations of outcomes are some elements that differentiate toughing out feared situations and useful exposure. Also, there can be strong divergence in the types of interventions offered by those claiming to offer cognitive-behavior therapy or exposure therapy. Just as one would never conclude medications don't work after trying one particular prescription, it does not make sense giving up on exposure therapy after trying one particular clinician.

By reviewing these misconceptions, we hope to communicate that exposure therapy can be delivered with all the richness and finesse that a clinician desires and that a patient needs. Exposure therapy can be added to any treatment where the clinician is comfortable taking a guiding role, helping patients learn what they do not know about psychopathology and the process of change. In exposure therapy, the clinician is a guide to teaching patients about some of the self-perpetuating patterns that characterize anxiety, its disorders, and their maintenance. Likewise, the clinician is a guide for showing patients how to approach phobic situations and events to be able to re-evaluate their relative safety. Finally, the clinician is a guide on how to process and consolidate these experiences to get the most out of exposure therapy.

1.2. The Art of "Playing" with Fear

It may be tempting for a clinician and patient to view reduced avoidance as an outcome that follows anxiety reduction rather than a primary therapeutic target in itself. Patients come to the clinic to feel better, and thus, to many, it feels counterintuitive to set up exercises that tackle avoidance head on and elicit fear and related emotions. Many clinicians are concerned that patients cannot tolerate the distress and/or translate these acts of courage during the session into meaningful improvements in symptoms. There is a sense that things can go badly, so why risk it? For example, one of our clinical trainees recently described her experience conducting prolonged exposure therapy with a new patient with posttraumatic stress disorder as stressful and draining. Seeing her patient upset when repeatedly recounting a memory of physical abuse had her wondering whether this exercise would really help the patient and prompted her to teach the patient a relaxation exercise instead. The patient welcomed the relaxation exercise as it matched her routine of fighting off fear, and the clinician left the session feeling reassured that she had done no harm.

This example is typical of our experience and reflects one of the challenges to conducting effective exposure therapy. In our own work in the clinic and the training of clinicians, we have found that exposure therapy becomes more appealing and effective when both clinicians and patients change their relationship with fear and related emotions as they arise during exposure therapy—from seeing distress as possibly problematic to viewing it as a positive signal for therapeutic learning. When you as clinicians trust that distress can be managed and that emotions are transient, you are in a better position to use exposure exercises as opportunities for new learning and consequent symptom improvement. When you believe fear activation signals that you are off to a good start, you can better model an adaptive response to distress. Instead of attempting to "rescue" the patient, you stay calm, offer support ("I know this is hard, but you are doing great"), and help the patient attend to and process the (safety) information that exposure exercises yield. In that way, you model the appropriate response to fear during exposure exercises: These emotional experiences reflect false alarms that, although producing discomfort, run their course when the patient and clinician act in ways that communicate that the patient is fine. Thus, an effective relationship with fear elicited during exposure therapy is evident when the clinician encourages the patient to embrace the discomfort ("anxiety is your green light; bring it on!"), helps them to resist the habitual avoidance and escape-oriented behaviors, and guides them to ride out the discomfort by doing "nothing."

Clinicians who trust that fear is an important part of the therapeutic process—those who are willing to "play with fear"—are less likely to hold back and therefore are better able to design and implement effective exposure exercises. Central to playing with fear is the development of a new relationship with the experience of anxiety. The anxiety signal becomes a herald for learning: It prompts an enquiring stance toward finding out what is accurate and what is false about this signal, and how this information can be used to enhance quality of life. Indeed, playing with fear implies that you (and the patient) are engaged and curious when you have found the (set of) cues that activate the patient's fear. And, when you (both) are excited that you have created the optimal circumstances for therapeutic learning, you can focus on getting the most out of this learning. That is, rather than attempting to provide comfort and immediate anxiety reduction, playing with fear means asking the patient to *lean into the feeling*, tolerating the moment, while attending to new information that contradicts fearful expectations. This book is dedicated to the many strategies that can be used to achieve these goals.

1.3. Personalized Exposure Therapy

We wrote this book to help make exposure therapy easier and more rewarding both for the patient and the clinician. It's true that, in many cases, simply guiding patients through a hierarchy of feared situations is all it takes to reduce fears. It's when such a manualized approach doesn't yield the desired effects that clinicians may be turned off by the method or question its efficacy. Being comfortable playing with fear is essential to achieving optimal outcomes quickly, as is personalizing exposure therapy.

The personalized approach to exposure therapy presented in this book stresses the importance of *case formulation.* That is, it encourages you to first work with your patient to develop an understanding of the factors that maintain fears for the patient. Complementing your clinical interviewing with self-report measures that assess thoughts and habits helps to

(1) determine the specific concerns—or appraisals of threat—driving the fears in situations; and
(2) identify the avoidance and escape maneuvers—or *safety behaviors*—that the patient uses to manage his or her fears (see Chapter 9 for a list of measures that can be used to assess these maintaining factors).

These two variables—threat appraisals and safety behaviors—are logically linked together, such that patients tend to adopt specific coping strategies that they believe will greatly reduce the perceived threat. Because they are idiosyncratic, these compensatory behaviors can be subtle and easily overlooked.

In addition to using the case formulation to fine-tune the exposure exercises to increase the salience and importance of the therapeutic learning—specifically setting up exposures that disconfirm fearful expectations—personalizing exposure therapy also means attending to individual differences in the processing of new information. Patients and clinicians easily align on treatment goals as determined during the intake process (e.g., reducing anxiety, enhancing self-esteem, increasing quality of life), yet they often think differently about the process required to achieve these goals. Most patients enter therapy thinking of their weekly therapy session as the hour for disclosure and support. Despite having an adequate discussion of the exposure therapy rationale, patients may not easily shift from seeing the session as an hour aimed at venting and feeling better to approaching it as an opportunity for safety learning. Indeed, as we describe in Chapter 4, entitled "Assessing Success," clinicians and patients may rate the value of the session using different criteria. Whereas the clinician will rate the session as successful when a patient recognizes that he or she overestimated perceived threats and is able to resist engaging in automated avoidance behaviors, a patient may rate session success by his or her sense of personal performance and anxiety level in an exposure practice. For example, we provide group treatment for social anxiety disorder that relies on repeated public speaking exposure exercises. We provide the rationale that repeated brief public speaking exposure exercises provide opportunities to respond differently to false alarms, allowing the fears to extinguish. Patients can articulate this model for therapeutic change—we know this because it is the topic of the first set of repeated speeches—but when processing the exposure exercises, many tend to focus on the quality of the speech. Patients who view the session as successful felt like they "nailed the speech." Their focus remains on becoming a better performer rather than being less concerned about performance. It is our job as clinicians to help these patients learn to view interim *therapeutic success* as having performed poorly without giving in to any of his automatic avoidance behaviors, thereby learning that the feared outcome (performing suboptimally) was actually manageable.

We believe that the degree to which a patient approaches the session as an opportunity for safety learning influences the rate of progress in exposure therapy. It is understandable when a patient feels relieved at the end of an exposure session—it takes a lot of energy to do the work. Yet, when this relief turns into avoiding the homework exposure exercises and the next in-session exercises, it is clear that adjustments need to be made in the patient's framing of exposure practice. In many cases, reframing is aided by a refocus on the exact learning goal for each exposure practice. The goal is not to "get through" the exposure, but to learn something specific from the experience of the exposure. Developing the right "dialogue" for this process is important. For example, a 33-year-old woman who presented with posttraumatic stress disorder in our clinic was able to articulate the treatment rationale for prolonged exposure therapy and showed excellent persistence in being able to repeatedly recount the memory of a rape that occurred when she was 27 years old. Yet, it wasn't until the clinician described exposure therapy as a method to help rearrange our "collage of memories of major life events" (reducing the size of the image representing the memory of the rape) that she started attending to the meaning of the memory (awful but not dangerous) during and following the sessions. Getting the dialogue right for your patient requires that you tell stories and provide metaphors that patients can relate to and, importantly, translate into the right action. We provide exemplar scripts throughout the book to aid you in this effort.

Therapeutic gains require learning during the session but obviously heavily depend on the extent to which patients retain or consolidate this new learning. It is striking to see the differences in the recounting of previous session experiences across patients. We are excited when we hear that a patient with fears of contamination reports that the experiences during the previous session prompted her to throw away all unnecessary cleaning agents—the exposure exercise during that session chipped away at the belief that contamination is harmful and deserving of the amount of attention she gives it. It is disheartening when the patient who evidenced a large reduction in the fear of fainting in a session that involved repeated practice with voluntary hyperventilation returns the following week to tell the clinician that he has started listening to a series of audio recordings that help him regulate his breathing (an obvious safety behavior in this case). Even though he recognized that the exposure session clearly demonstrated that feeling faint does not lead to fainting, this new learning did not cement into useful awareness.

It may be fair to assume that most patients generally make good use of what they learn during a session, but the example of the patient presenting with a fear of fainting underscores the importance of attending to take-away messages. For this patient, the clinician may complement the end of session review of what he learned during the session with a discussion focused on how to translate this learning into real-life behavioral change. This discussion becomes the basis of specific homework exercises (e.g., journaling, discussing the exercise with a friend/partner, repetition of the exposure exercise at home) designed to make the learning stick.

1.4. How to Use This Book

Our focus for this book is on the principles and procedures that guide exposure therapy; this is a "how to" book. We further break this information into the specific steps you can take to prepare for and implement sessions, with lots of practical information that you can quickly review before starting a session. For many of the procedures, we provide scripts that you can use or easily adapt into the "language" you feel most comfortable using with your patients. The book is also full of figures, worksheets, and handouts that can be used during the session. To make it easier for you, we have made key materials available on a website that complements this text (www.oup.com/us/personalizedexposure). We seriously considered providing in-text citations, as this is the standard approach to giving credit to the people who have done the work informing this book. We ended up deciding to forego in-text citations, simply because we were concerned that doing so would result in another more technical and thus possibly less accessible and appealing book on how to deliver exposure therapy. We want to be clear though that the ideas that we present in this book have very much been shaped by the research conducted by our mentors, peers, and students as well as the conversations in clinical supervision with our fellow clinicians and trainees. We acknowledge several of them throughout the book and have provided a list of key references in the bibliography section.

The first section of the book, Chapters 2 to 4, provides a framework for conducting personalized exposure therapy. Specifically, Chapter 2 offers a "forest instead of the trees" overview of principles behind exposure therapy and the way in which new learning is integrated in memory structures. In short, we use a memory-centric view of exposure therapy that is designed to help clinicians identify what is likely to be learned from individual exposure sessions, and how to arrange exposures to provide fuller safety learning. Chapter 3 translates Chapter 2 into the general approach to conducting exposure therapy (i.e., how to implement it), highlighting case formulation, the principles of delivering exposure exercises, and the techniques that help ensure that the patient gets the most out of the session. Chapter 4 complements Chapter 3 by guiding you how to make decisions about treatment progression as it introduces "yardsticks" for improvement that you can use to determine whether you and your patient are on track.

The second section of the book, Chapters 5 to 8, describes the application of personalized exposure therapy to the core fear cues evident across anxiety and related disorders—emotions and physical sensations (Chapter 5), people (Chapter 6), thoughts, images, and traumatic memories (Chapter 7)—and discusses specific strategies for how to combine exposure therapy with medications (Chapter 8).

The third and last section of the book, Chapters 9 to 11, provides you with additional resources, including a list of assessment of strategies (Chapter 9), materials for patient education (Chapter 10), and some of the key references to research papers, chapters, and books that have informed the approach to exposure therapy that we discuss in this book (Chapter 11).

2

Thinking Through Exposure

No two patients are the same. Hence, being effective with exposure therapy requires making adjustments depending on how the patient presents and how she responds to your interventions. Thinking on your feet becomes easy when you have a framework for how to be effective with exposure therapy—a clear idea of what you're aiming to accomplish and an awareness of factors that either facilitate or impede these goals. This chapter provides a conceptual model for understanding the persistence of fear responses and the ways in which exposure therapy can be tasked to creating stronger safety memories.

2.1. Fear as a Set of Memories

As we have noted, exposure therapy is not a passive weakening of learned fear associations. Instead it is the active relearning of safety in relation to feared cues. And like any new learning, this learning has to be recalled in the moments of life where it is relevant to be useful. Accordingly, one element of successful therapy for anxiety disorders is the creation of memories of relative safety that guide adaptive functioning and minimize distress.

Fear memories are complex. They engender the outcome expectancies, emotions, and escape and avoidance responses that define anxiety disorders. Fear memories are also encoded at two levels:

(1) A direct series of cue-based associations that define the meaning of cues in terms of danger expectations.
(2) Verbal abstractions of these cues.

Correctly executed exposure therapy intervenes at both of these levels of encoding—lower-order associative processes as well as higher-order conceptual learning—to help patients relearn a sense of safety in response to fear cues. That is, exposure therapy provides experience for reshaping associations between cues and outcomes and for reforming rules about the dangerousness of these cues. To achieve both of these outcomes efficiently, exposure therapy needs to engage patients cognitively, with attention to how patients conceptualize each exposure and its outcome.

One crucial feature of fear and safety memories is that one does not simply replace the other. Instead, fear and safety memories can be in competition. The resolution of this competition—in terms of older fear memories or therapy-related safety memories—determines clinical outcome and the likelihood of relapse. Hence, one goal of exposure therapy is to create especially salient safety memories that, because of the way in which they have been integrated with relevant cues, win the competition over fear memories in terms of shaping functioning. Accordingly, we believe that knowing how fear and safety memories are likely to interact can enhance exposure planning and the achievement of a long-lasting treatment response.

As we all know well, experiences don't simply replace one another in memory. Instead, new experiences are integrated into existing memory structures to update them, strengthening redundant information and refining memory relative to new information. To help understand this process, picture the structure of a memory as a network of interconnected nodes; the elements of a memory depend on the strength and type of connectivity between the nodes of cues/meaning, and, quite reasonably, related memories have overlapping neuronal clusters in their respective networks of connectivity.

To update a memory, the nature of the connections can be strengthened or changed. In many cases, new information is added while keeping the original memory intact. In essence, the new memory becomes a special case or a refined aspect of the old memory. A memory of a happy dog can sit side by side with a memory of a growling dog. Both are true, and which memory comes up depends on which other cues are activated (e.g., white dogs growl; brown dogs nuzzle).

As more memories are added, more global attributes about a cue may dominate the special cases (dogs are mostly scary, but some dogs are OK), or a memory may be so salient or so frequently rehearsed that the older memory is changed to accommodate this new information (all dogs are scary). An important corollary to this process is that memories are not fixed at the moment of the experience but are activated and once again become malleable after we recall a memory. This malleability is thought to be a natural process of refining the memory. We do not recall the same memory again and again over time. Instead, we repeatedly recall modified memories that are active reconsolidations of older memories.

2.1.1. The Structure of Memories: An Example

To provide a fuller accounting of memory change, let's consider an example outside the realm of fear. When a friend treats you poorly at lunch, you have to integrate this experience with everything else you know about your friend. If you have lots of positive experiences with your friend, John, this new behavior will stand as an aberration and may well be encoded as a special case ("John is a nice guy, but sometimes he may exhibit surprising and not very pleasant behavior"). But if there are repetitions of John's bad behavior, negative associations to John will be strengthened and may form an alternative set of competing memory to the original conceptualization of John as a nice guy. This is a core feature of adapting to changing circumstances: Two sets of memories are competing, those associated with pleasurable lunches and those associated with John treating you poorly. Accordingly, your emotional expectancies for lunch will depend on which set of memories (pleasant or aversive) are dominant when you are next cued by John's face at the lunch table. The memories are in competition.

Of course, there are things you can do to bias which memories are most salient (are most likely to win the competition for your dominant expectancies). You may, for example, conceptually rewrite the story of the friendship ("It just isn't worth it to be friends with John") or to rewrite the conceptualization of what you think of your friend as a person ("John is a jerk"). You may come to this new conceptualization on your own, or it may occur as you get input from someone else ("You know, you often feel this way after lunch with John, I don't know why you think he is such a good friend"). This *postevent reprocessing* of what happened at lunch and its meaning likely will be retained along with the latest lunch experience. The memory, slowly consolidated over several hours, represents the integration of the *experience* and the active *interpretation of the experience* within the existing clusters of nodes (neuronal connections) that form the memory of "John at lunch."

The strength of a new, more negative memory of John should depend on:

(1) The salience of the negative experience.
(2) The salience of the negative rehearsal of the experience after the event.
(3) The degree to which both can be seen as typical of John.

That is, if John's negative behavior occurs under unusual circumstance (e.g., as part of a three-martini lunch), it may take much more postevent processing to generalize expectancies around "jerk John" versus the assimilation of a unique memory of "John while intoxicated." In sum, new and old memories are linked (integrated) relative to the degree to which they have shared attributes.

To learn from ongoing experiences is to alter our memories of our experiences so that we have either a more nuanced (and hopefully more accurate) set of expectancies about what will happen upon subsequent exposure to a cue. Figures 2.1 through 2.4 exemplify these processes. In Figure 2.1, the assimilation of novel and negative information about John is illustrated by a tentative

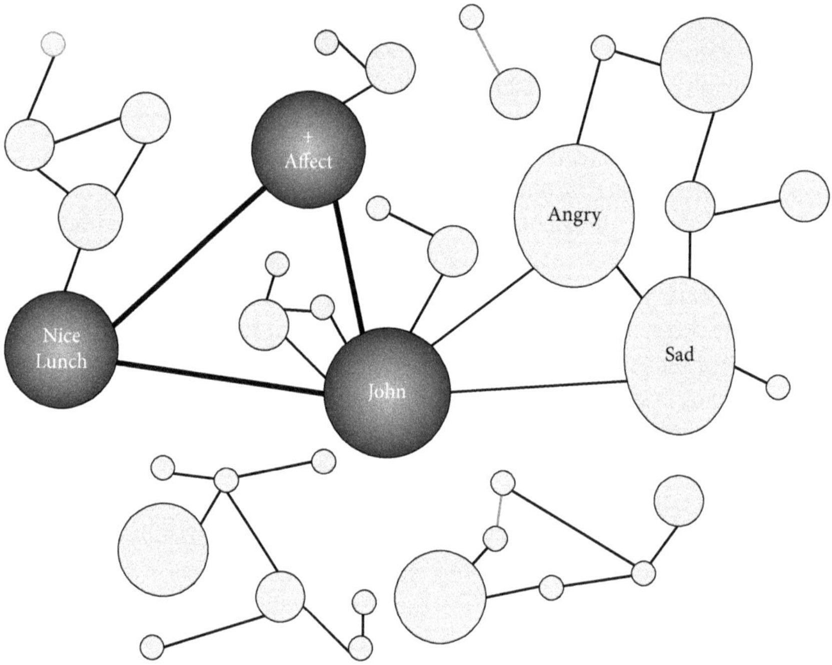

Figure 2.1 Nodes of the novel memory of an aversive lunch with John. Node model adapted from Landsman et al. (2014). The reorganisation of memory during sleep. *Sleep Medicine Review, 18*, 5315–5341.

and weak link to negative affectivity. With multiple repetitions, that link will be strengthened to provide a stronger negative association to John that competes with the original positive memories of John (Figure 2.2). The negative memories may be further strengthened by links to the broader concepts of "people who are not nice," adding additional negative emotional salience to expectancies around John (Figure 2.3). Finally, in Figure 2.4, there is the tentative integration of contextual information that may differentiate "nice John" from "jerk John"—the presence of way too much vodka.

The natural conflict between the two sets of expectancies about John may lead to active attempts to resolve the dissonance between the perspectives. In other words, you may set up a test of your views of John to see which is correct. Prior to meeting John for lunch, for example, you may review (activate) each conceptualization (each set of memories and expectations) about John and then intentionally evaluate which set of expectancies best fits your upcoming experiences during lunch. If John treats you badly only when he drinks, this contextual information will gain value in shaping your expectancies of which version of John will

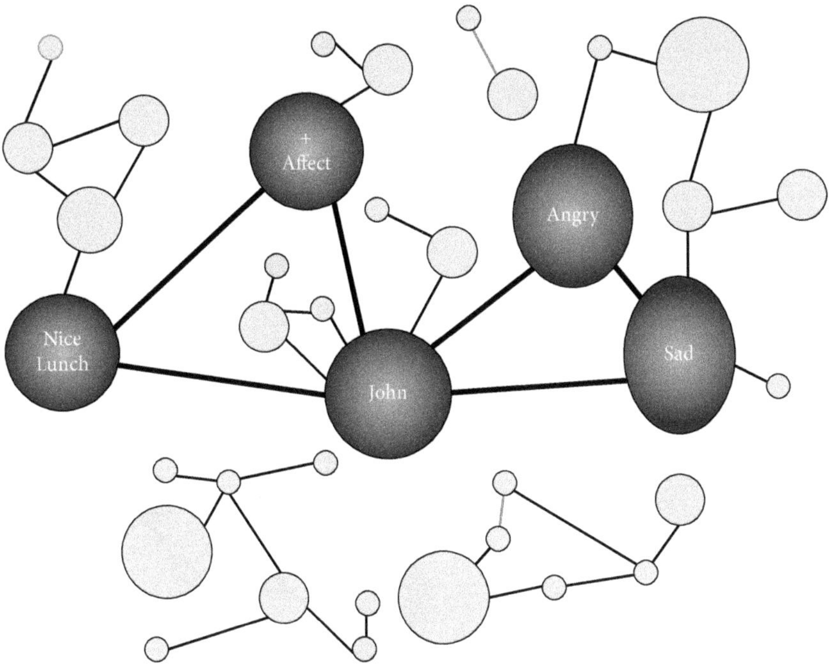

Figure 2.2 Competition between positive and negative memories of lunch with John.

emerge. But if he treats you badly in multiple contexts (drinking or not, under job stress or not), you may resolve the conflict in expectancies more globally—John is a jerk. That evaluation would then be part of the reconsolidated memory evoked by the complex set of cues that is John.

It is interesting to consider whether the lunch-time evaluative "test" of John is an example of exposure therapy or cognitive therapy. It certainly draws from traditions of each. Concerning exposure therapy, a focused experience is used to resolve the ambiguous meaning of a cue (John). The test involved preactivation of two sets of expectations and relied on planned vigilance to resolve the discrepancies by attentively observing the experience at hand, with strengthening of the learning by reviewing and rehearsing what was learned at the conclusion of the test. Concerning cognitive therapy, the evaluative test of John involves the active monitoring of cognitions that may or may not reflect common distortions held by the patient. In relation to these cognitions, ongoing situations are then evaluated to see if an alternative conceptualization of events may be apt. Both cognitive therapy and exposure therapy hone the patient's ability to "see beyond expectancies," to

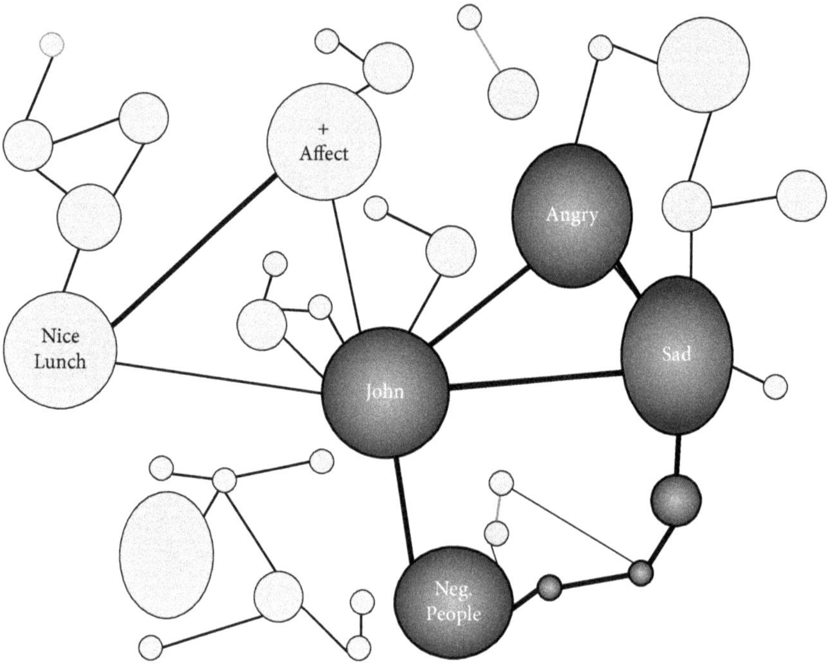

Figure 2.3 Negative memories of John come to dominate and are integrated with the concept of "people who are not nice."

evaluate events more objectively, and to use the resulting information to actively shift future expectancies. Learning occurs at both the level of experiential (associative) learning and at the level of cognitive monitoring, rehearsal, and integration.

Schema activation is a concept relevant to both cognitive therapy and exposure therapy models. From a memory-science perspective, the ease with which new learning about John is consolidated is influenced by how well this new learning fits existing schemas. That is, people learn new information more easily when memory structures already provide a "landing zone" for this information. For example, the ease with which a person sees John as having changed for the worse depends in part on whether there is a ready-made schema for a shift of this kind. Previous learning may have established a "People sometimes change for the worse" memory structure that can be subsequently attached to John, allowing for drawing on these experiences to make sense out of John's behavior. The greater the number of experiences of having a friendship go bad, the more easily John and his negative behavior may be consolidated into strong negative expectancies. There is an important principle at work here: The integration of a novel memory

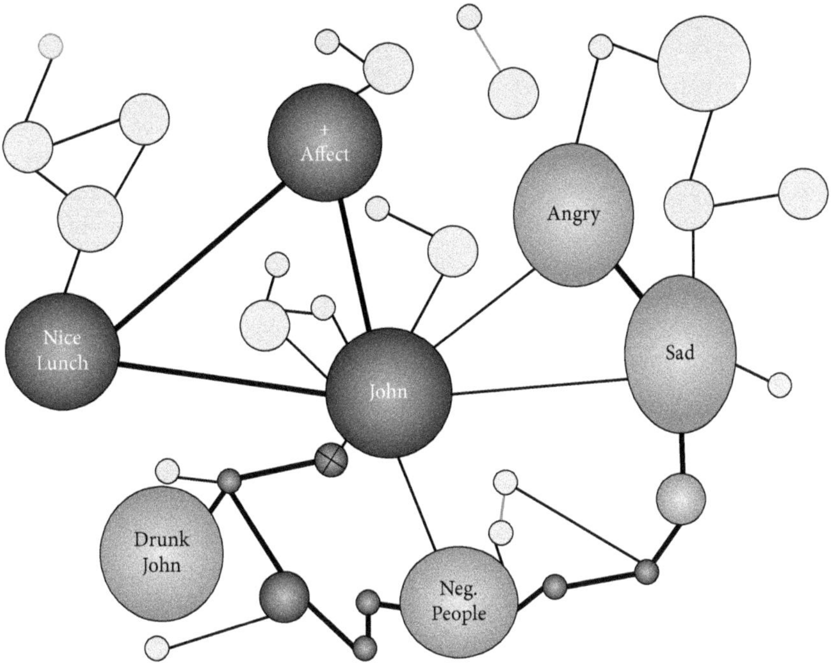

Figure 2.4 Integration of contextual information for the aversiveness of John at lunch.

is aided by a "landing zone" for that memory—a pre-existing schema that aids the interpretation and integration of the experienced events. Such schematic landing zones aid the consolidation of new memories and, indeed, may bias the content of these memories.

With the strengthening of a negative view of John, what then happens to the earlier memories of nice John? The salience of these memories may be weakened, but the memories do not disappear. Instead, they may be relegated to their own context. Time is one such powerful context. For all sorts of shifts in the meaning of stimuli, we use a version of "That was then; this is now" to make sense of the new reality. For example, "I used to be a bad dancer in high school, but now I know my moves" or "I was a C student in high school, but in college I found my mark" are both ways to summarize our expectancies for shifts in personal performance that occur over time. With such time-based or development-based distinctions, we drop our allegiance to the long-past and allow ourselves to be better shaped by our experience from the recent-past. As said by L. P. Hartley, "the past is a foreign country; they do things differently there." We fathom the true meaning of cues by updating memories.

2.1.2. Context and Expectancy

If we were to try to predict how you would react emotionally to seeing John at a particular lunch (which memories and thereby which expectancies), we would have to know about your broader history with John, your broader history with being treated poorly by friends, and about lots of state factors that serve as links to either "nice John" or "jerk John" memories. For example, a demeaning experience earlier in the day may set off mood-state dependent links to "jerk John" memories, because of the way in which negative mood is linked to "jerk John" memories (as illustrated in Figure 2.5). As such, a wide variety of contextual factors—your mood, your level of stress, the amount of sleep you had, whether your drive to lunch was easy or frustrating, and the color shirt you are wearing—can serve to activate different sets of memories about John, depending on their match to the contextual factors at the time of encoding and consolidation, which means that to understand the reliability of a particular set of expectations about John, one has to understand all the factors that may influence which set of expectations will be evoked. For example, even if during your morning shower you coach yourself that "John has been a good friend for years, I am sure that lunch will go well and that I will have a good time," during the mid-morning you may

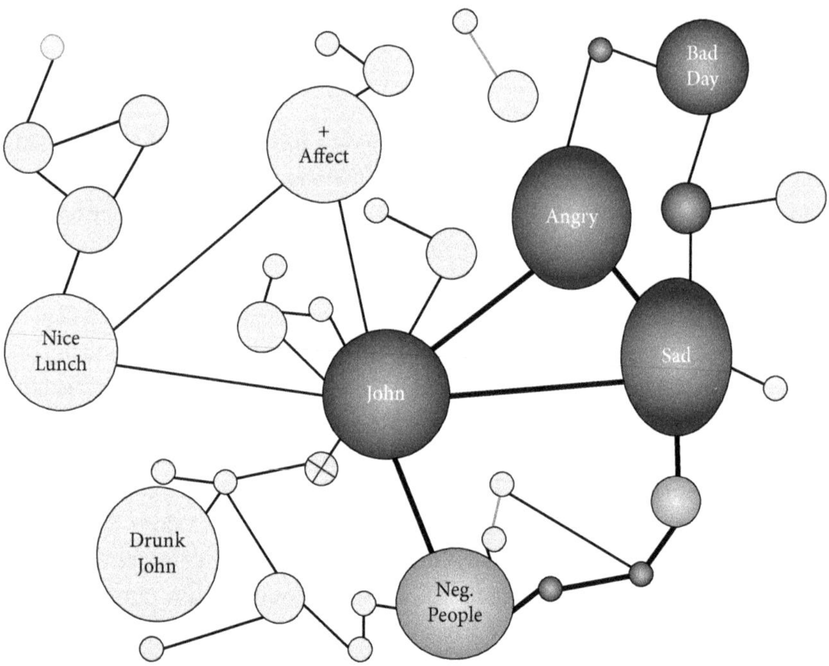

Figure 2.5 A negative experience cues negative expectancies of John at lunch.

be buffeted by a number of contextual cues of the bad lunches with John, cueing an increased sense of foreboding about lunch.

Memories that are context-specific can easily be retained, despite alternative experiences, until such a time that a dominant memory is formed across contexts. How does this arise? Direct experiences across contexts or memory rehearsals across contexts help generalize the learning—creating a truly cross-context expectancy. As Meghan Trainor sings, "My name is no, my sign is no, my number is no. You need to let it go. You need to let it go." Consistency across contexts provides a resilient and less assailable expectancy.

2.2. The Structure of Fear Memories and Its Implications for Exposure Therapy

This simple example of learning new expectancies for John-at-lunch has some clear implications for the process of exposure therapy/safety learning that is essential to good clinical outcomes. With effective exposure therapy, clinicians are actively shaping patients' expectations about feared cues—creating new memories (new expectations) of safety relative to these cues. As with any other sort of memory formation, clinicians need to be concerned with providing salient learning opportunities that are relevant to the fear cues as well as the contexts that further define the threat associated with these cues. As such, maximizing adaptive learning from exposure can then be translated into the degree that exposure provides

(1) An adequate match to the cues that define a patient's fears.
(2) Adequate attention to the contexts that modulate the degree of fear.
(3) A strong and unambiguous disconfirmation of threat expectancies associated with the fear cue.
(4) The degree of active interpretation and rehearsal of the meaning of the event after the exposure experience.

Let's consider each of these factors in turn.

2.2.1. The Degree of Match to Fear Cues

The entire idea of a hierarchy of exposure sessions (proceeding from moderate levels of fear to high levels of fear) reflects the importance of ultimately achieving a strong match between the exposure experiences and the patient's expectancies of threat. The goal is to update the meaning of these threat cues, so that they no longer signal fear and avoidance. To update the meaning of the fear stimuli, the clinician provides sequential learning and frequent rehearsal of safety in response to these cues. The degree of match is defined by effective assessment and validated by a patient's anticipatory anxiety during exposure planning. The match need not be defined by high anxiety *during exposure itself.* The degree of anxiety during exposure is a product of both the pre-existing expectations of harm (which are high as determined during assessment) and the subsequent in-exposure assessments of threat (which the clinician wants to demonstrate to be low). Low anxiety during exposure may be an especially good sign of progress, as long as there are no other factors that invalidate the meaning of the fear cues (see Chapter 4). Let's turn next to potential invalidating contexts.

2.2.2. Contexts

The contexts in which fear cues are encountered can enhance or degrade the meaning of these cues. As such, contexts can determine the scope of benefit of an exposure session. If there is a strong match between the context and the patient's expectancies of fear, there is a strong potential for useful safety learning. Yet, if the context defines the exposure session as occurring due to special and unique circumstances, safety learning may be encoded alongside current fear-memory networks and do little to offer the patient reliable benefit. Such derailing contexts are sometimes defined by the presence of safety cues or safety behaviors. We devote major attention to safety behaviors in the chapters that follow, but, in short, they include behaviors and cues that communicate that a threat was reduced during an exposure because of the safety cue. Safety cues include such things as the presence of anxiety-rescue medicines (e.g., benzodiazepine), the clinician ("She will help me"), cell phones ("I can call my spouse for help"), time of day (exposures during a sunny day may feel very different than exposures during a dark winter evening), and safety behaviors such as tensing up muscles to prevent untoward actions, breathing deeply, or averting one's eyes. Safety cues can also include more durable contexts such as being on antidepressant medications, feeling rested, feeling emotionally connected to a spouse, or in a low-stress phase at work. Contexts can moderate the meaning of the exposure session; the job of the clinician is to work to extend safety learning across multiple contexts by either conducting exposure across relevant contexts or by working to help the patient generalize their experiences across the contexts.

Given the ubiquity of circumstances and events that can serve as a safety cue, the onus is on the clinician to remain vigilant to and assess the presence of safety cues. As we make clear in subsequent chapters, what a clinician does about safety cues evolves across treatment. Early sessions of exposure are devoted to providing initial learning of safety, and safety cues may be richly present during this initial learning. Yet, for fuller learning of safety (and prevention of relapse due to context shifts), safety behaviors and cues are more actively targeted in later sessions. This can be thought of as its own progression along a hierarchy. In early exposure sessions learning of safety may be conditional ("I can face my fears . . . as long as my clinician is with me, I have my cell phone and bottle of water, and I have my pills in my pocket"), in later sessions it is broad based ("I can face my fear on a bad day and even with no preparation"). As summarized nicely by Michael Telch and colleagues,

> Safety behaviors should be used sparingly, and introduced early in the treatment in order to reduce dropouts and increase the patient's sense of control and confidence. Safety behaviors can also be introduced later in therapy as a way to assist the patient in overcoming specific obstacles encountered during the course of treatment. Based on the consistent evidence [for impairing effects on safety learning], it is suggested that clinicians pay careful attention to the fading of safety behaviors over the course of treatment. The fading of safety behaviors not only enhances the patient's sense of mastery but also reduces the chance that patients will misattribute their success to the aid rather than their own efforts.

In subsequent chapters, we provide additional strategies for assessing safety behaviors, but, in general, cross-context learning as well as safety cue assessments can be elucidated by close questioning about what was learned from a specific exposure. These questions take two forms. In the general form, patients are simply asked what they "make of their exposure experiences." This corresponds, in our example about John, to a question like "What did you make of John's behavior today at lunch?" The purpose is to aid active evaluation and broad consolidation of exposure success. In a specific form of these questions, the patient is asked specifically about why a feared outcome *did not* occur. This corresponds, in the example about John, to a direct test of the expectancies regarding his behavior: "Why do you think John continued to act badly today?" If the answer is context specific, the clinician has a chance to challenge that interpretation or, more powerfully, to plan a subsequent exposure that eliminates that conditional context. This process is aided by an active regeneration of these expectancies and context-specific interpretations ("In last week's exposure, you thought that you might have done well just because I was with you; this week we will test that hypothesis by having you conduct similar exposures without me").

These questions about context-specific interpretations of safety learning are a special case of the importance of postexposure processing—the active review of what was learned from exposure practice. Postevent processing of exposure practice is aimed at highlighting discrepancies between the patient's fearful expectations and what actually occurred. To achieve this goal, clinicians have to have a clear definition of which outcomes signify a violation of fearful expectations and which do not. For these reasons, we now turn to the crucial topic of evaluation of outcomes.

2.2.3. Evaluation of Outcome

What constitutes a threat-free outcome in exposure therapy? The answer lies in the eye of the beholder. Which is to say, there are many subjective outcomes that are idiosyncratically feared by patients. These subjective outcomes occur in addition to the obvious perceived threats associated with fears, phobias, and the anxiety disorders: Perceived dangerous outcomes such as falling from high places, having a trauma recur, having a stroke during panic, being contaminated by dangerous germs, injuring a loved one, or becoming a social pariah. What are the additional concerns or threat appraisals? They often not only have to do with catastrophic interpretations of the signs and symptoms of anxiety itself (e.g., feeling anxious, trembling, flushing, or sweating) but may also include social outcomes such as becoming embarrassed, doing something foolish, or making mistakes. These latter concerns are perceived as catastrophic but are not, and safety learning relative to these outcomes often focuses not on the nonoccurrence of these events, but on the relative unimportance of the occurrence of these events. This distinction deserves careful attention and a clear definition:

(1) There are fears associated with true dangers and are resolved by helping patients understand the routine nonoccurrence of these dangers.
(2) There are fears of relatively innocuous events, and these fears may be resolved by either attention to the rare elicitation of these events, the innocuous survivability of these events, or a combination of these factors.

If this distinction sounds familiar, it is because it maps well onto the two cognitive distortions identified in the field as ubiquitous to the anxiety and worry-based disorders:

(1) The overestimation of the probability of negative outcomes—or *likelihood bias*.
(2) The overestimation of the degree of the catastrophe of these outcomes—or *cost bias*.

For the former concerns, corrective information is aimed at showing these outcomes do not occur frequently enough to justify the fear. For the latter perceived threats, corrective information is targeted to understanding the survivability of these feared outcomes.

In planning exposure assignments, these two types of fears cannot be confused. Part of the job of the clinician is to help the patient define what are acceptable outcomes from exposure: When the explicit goal is the nonoccurrence of a feared outcome as compared to when the explicit goal is the enhanced tolerability to the occurrence of feared outcome. For most anxiety and worry-related disorders, part of therapeutic learning is the learning that the experience of anxiety itself is tolerable. This learning involves the distinction between the experience of anxiety and feared negative outcomes such as loss of control, social rejection, failure, or impending harm. Part of this learning may come from observing the time course of anxiety symptoms ("You know, my anxiety is really bad for a few minutes and then decreases" or "My anxiety comes in waves, sometimes at unexpected moments"), and sometimes this anxiety comes from monitoring and learning the distinction between the experience of anxiety and objective outcomes by remaining in feared situations long enough to observe goal consequences. For example, Rick Heimberg, in his group treatment of social anxiety disorder, suggests that in treatment patients first learn that they meet their social interactional goals despite the presence of anxiety and then, subsequently, have their anxiety dissipate in the context of repeated evidence of relative social success. In short, patients learn that their experience of anxiety is not as predictive of their social outcomes as they assumed, and, once this principle is learned, patients can focus their social interactions on maximizing their desired social outcomes.

For other disorders, learning safety in the context of anxiety symptoms is specifically programmed rather than incidental and is a major component of treatment. In the treatment of panic disorder, for example, interoceptive exposure procedures (see Chapter 5) are used to directly teach alternative (safety) conceptualizations of the meaning of anxiety symptoms. Regardless of which of these strategies is utilized, anxiety is a regular companion on the road to recovery, and, accordingly, learning relative comfort to these symptoms is an early goal for exposure treatment. For this reason, care has to be taken in exposure planning to help ensure that the experience of anxiety itself does not define a failure experience in exposure.

Yet, anxiety reduction or elimination is a goal for every anxiety patient. Treatment certainly is aimed at anxiety reduction, but *full elimination* of anxiety is not a goal that is readily commiserate with active engagement in life. Life involves anxiety, and, as such, a fallback goal for individuals desiring an elimination of anxiety is a reframing this goal to changing one's relationship with anxiety—to reduce both the aversiveness of the experience of anxiety and to reduce ways in which anxiety interferes with value-driven action. As such, treatment involves a refinement of treatment goals toward those that reflect an understanding of anxiety's function as a true alarm, a false alarm, and a feared outcome in itself. Anxiety's function as a true alarm (as a harbinger of true or legitimate threat) is to be respected; anxiety's function as a false alarm (as a false signal of the presence of threat) is to be treated using exposure to show that feared outcomes do not follow anxious expectations; and anxiety's function as feared outcome in itself is to be treated by enhancing tolerability of these sensations.

These different meanings of anxiety and corresponding targets of exposure mean that treatment involves an active translation of ultimate treatment goals (reduced anxiety and disability) to any of a number of interim treatment goals, sometimes in a paradoxical way. For example, for the treatment of panic disorder—a disorder characterized by the patient's rightful and overwhelming desire to quash anxiety and panic episodes—treatment is focused on reducing the fear of panic symptoms as a necessary first goal. When elimination of the fear of panic is achieved, so too is elimination of the regular elicitation of panic attacks. Thus, clinicians have to translate the goal of being panic free to an interim goal of not fearing panic. Likewise, in the treatment of social anxiety disorder, patients may enter treatment with a desperate desire to avoid embarrassment or any social act that may be interpreted as "weird, faulty, or abnormal." Given the ubiquity of such acts, it is not desperate avoidance of these acts that is a good goal, but acceptance that these events are normal and lead to very few adverse consequences. Accordingly, clinicians may need to translate goals of relative social invulnerability into interim goals of being more accepting of and comfortable with social gaffs, minor embarrassment, and anxiety symptoms. Indeed, the evocation of purposeful social gaffs in exposures (i.e., social cost exposures; see Chapter 6) is designed to enhance social comfort, not by avoiding these outcomes, but by showing these outcomes do not have serious consequences.

Again, clinicians need to translate the patient's ultimate goals of social comfort into the relevant learning events. Developing the ability to endure social comfort may progress along the following continuum of therapeutic learning of fuller and fuller social safety. For example, one characteristic of socially anxious individuals is the assumption that observers are better than they are at identifying anxiety symptoms experienced by the individual. As such, the subjective experience of anxiety may be defined as evidence of social rejection, and conditional safety can be defined as:

- Limited safety—If I don't have anxiety symptoms, I think I will be OK socially.

- Partial safety—Others do not seem to notice my anxiety symptoms (there are no social consequences), so I don't need to worry about making a fool out of myself.
- Fuller safety—Even if others notice my anxiety symptoms, it does not mean that I am making a fool out of myself or that I will be socially rejected.

The transition across these definitions of safety is determined by the degree of inclusion of induced anxiety symptoms within the social exposures, changing the type of safety learning targeted. Likewise, the following examples represent a transition to greater social safety as social gaffs are programmed into the social exposure practice:

- Limited safety—If I don't make a mistake, I think I will be OK socially.
- Partial safety—Others do not seem to notice my minor gaffs (there are no social consequences), so I don't need to worry about making a fool out of myself.
- Fuller safety—Even if I make clear gaffs, it does not mean that I will be socially rejected.

It is true that none of us are eager to have multiple social gaffs, and purposeful social gaff exposures may bear only limited resemblance to the ultimate goal of greater social ease. Nonetheless, the creation of safety around these gaffs, should they occur, creates broad-based changes to vigilance and monitoring of potential gaffs, thereby decreasing anxiety and enhancing social ease. In leading patients through exposures like these, the clinician provides a patient with information on the most useful "yardstick" by which to measure progress in each phase of therapy, depending on what types of fears are targeted. Once targets and outcomes are identified, both clinician and patient cheer on progress toward this yardstick in the context of individual exposure sessions (see also Chapter 4).

To review, exposure therapy utilizes very different targets for fears depending on whether they represent an exaggerated probability of negative outcomes or an exaggerated sense of catastrophe of outcomes. For the former, exposure tracks the *nonoccurrence* of the anticipated feared event, and for the latter, exposure tracks the learning of *safety despite the occurrence* of the feared event. Which type of corrective learning needs to be applied depends on the particular threats idiosyncratically defined by each patient as well as the stage of treatment. Should learning that anxiety symptoms themselves do not confer danger come before or after learning that the feared events that evoke anxiety are an overestimation of threat? The answer to this question lies in the patient's own hierarchy of fears and the degree by which anxiety is defined as a feared outcome in itself. Because anxiety is so frequently a consequence of exposure, if anxiety is itself a feared outcome, it makes sense to intervene first to reduce the aversiveness of anxiety. Otherwise, both patient and clinicians may spin their wheels in therapy.

2.2.4. Helping Patients Attend to What Was Learned

The task of generalizing exposure safety learning is strengthened on pre- and postexposure processing, in addition to clear definitions and evaluations of feared outcomes. We now turn to the importance of clear definitions of outcome. Box 2.1 includes some generic questions that clinicians might use to help them clarify their expectancies and to hone their outcome evaluations prior to exposure. With their expectancies clarified, patients are well-prepared to integrate new memories into their current fear structures.

Box 2.1 Postexposure Processing Questions

Opening Questions

- Well, tell me how that went from your perspective?
- How did you do? Did you meet your goals for that exposure?
- If we keep in mind that exposure is a chance to learn something new about a fear cue, what did you learn from this exposure?

Questions to Cue Attention to Expectancy Violations

- How did your experience differ from what you expected?
- When you think back, what were you expecting before this exposure? How did you experiences match or differ from this expectation?
- As compared to what you were thinking before this exposure, how might you coach yourself differently for your next exposure?

Questions to Cue Generalization Strategies

- How can you best sum up what was valuable about today's exposure practices?
- If you were going to provide guidance to someone else with fears like yours, what would you say to her about what you learned from this exposure?
- What in particular do you want to remember about this session over the next week?
- How can what you apply what you have learned today over the next week?

There is initial evidence that the benefits of exposure are better maintained when the patient is in (or is induced to be in) a better mood at the time of (before, during, and after) exposure. One way to understand this effect is that a positive mood is an emotional cue that is generally incompatible with threat. Accordingly, incorporating a positive mood in the exposure memory provides a potentially powerful interpretive link for the new safety memories. Also, positive affectivity may reduce subtle avoidance behaviors linked to anxiety and allow a greater depth of processing of the exposure experience. Two strategic considerations for exposure therapy follow from this accounting. First, use of humor in exposure therapy is a tool not only to aid adherence by breaking the tension of the session, but it also has implications for setting in a more powerful safety memory. That is, it is not unusual for expert behavior clinicians to mention the ways in which they use quips, turns of phrases, or self-deprecating humor when introducing or leading a patient toward exposure therapy. This humor, specifically the memory of feeling relatively light-hearted when exposure is initiated may provide a useful memory to help patient get past the reticence and avoidance common for home practice assignments.

A more important consideration, though, is the conceptualization of exposure therapy that is not simply anxiety reduction but is well-being enhancement. The ultimate goal of exposure therapy is the recreation of pleasure in the presence of threat cues. Consider an assignment for agoraphobia that asks a patient to go to the mall as part of an exposure assignment to learn safety by staying in the mall until her anxiety has an opportunity to dissipate. Now consider an exposure assignment that asks a patient to actively window shop, people-watch, and enjoy the feeling of being out in the world, while also allowing her anxiety to dissipate with the experience of being there. Both rationales encourage exposure, but the latter strategy also provides a better frame for positive affect before, during, and after the formal exposure. This frame likewise creates a more positive association with the fear cues (moments of joy in the mall), which have the potential to speed recovery and provide a stronger bulwark against relapse. These positive memories are also likely to help with avoidance of exposure assignments; exposure will feel like less work when there are positive memories and positive agendas linked to the assignments. Indeed, one of the goals of treatment is to re-establish normal and functional behaviors in the presence of fear cues. Attending to the joys of situational exposures helps define this return to normal, not just nonphobic, behavior and, hence, should be a considered part of exposure programming.

2.3. Learning to Learn

One of the early tasks of exposure therapy is to help patients develop the schema that treatment—specifically, exposure to feared cues—is helpful. There are a number of elements to this learning. First, there is early learning on how to approach exposure assignments with an attentive mind. Specifically, this attentive mind involves a readiness to observe and notice the difference between (a) expectations about what is going to happen and (b) what actually happens. This learning is aided by programmed practice attending to various aspects of a feared situation. Shifting attention alone may be a challenge for some patients, reflecting the degree of automaticity that their fear responses (hypervigilance to specific coping/superstitious responses) have achieved over time. Shifting this attention is important for evaluating the true nature of exposure outcomes. For example, there is evidence that vigilance to safety cues can hinder processing of the absence of threats in an exposure situation (e.g., repeatedly checking for the presence of a pill in the pocket draws attention from fully noticing the relative safety of the feared event). Likewise, the work of David Clark and colleagues shows that self-focused attention, as compared to situation- or other-focused attention, hinders adaptive safety learning from exposure. Self-focused attention ensures that negative self-evaluations and the anxiety symptoms can play a more central role in biasing the evaluation of the true safety of the situation. Accordingly, the first phase of exposure learning involves learning how to accurately approach and attend to the exposure situation.

Second, early learning sets the stage for less strongly held expectancies around the feared cues. In terms of our model of lunch with John, an aberrant lunch experience occasions a broader evaluation of John, setting up initial competition between new and old expectancies of how lunch will go. Likewise, initial exposure experiences can provide a new and disparate meaning of fear cues that can then be used in a broader test of core fears. Initial learning from exposure may be as simple as "It does not always go the way I fear" or "Depending on what I pay attention to, I have a different experience." There are likely strong context effects for this new learning, where any safety learning is dependent on the unique context of the presence of the clinician and the specific exposure instructions and practices that were undertaken. This context specificity is nonetheless useful for establishing initial ambivalence about the meaning of fear cues, introducing the memory that "I can do/feel better in this treatment." There are two core advantages to such learning. First, it provides initial evidence contradicting fear expectancies that is then used as part of preparation for subsequent exposures: "Let's bring to mind your expectations about how this exposure will go. In the past you have assumed that . . . , but more recently you found that . . ." Second, it provides initial learning that exposure can work, creating a useful schema by which to approach and integrate subsequent more difficult exposure experiences. In terms of the memory model previously explicated, early sessions are devoted to creating an "exposure works" memory node, thereby establishing a useful landing zone for subsequent expectations and successes with exposure. More broadly, as memories of exposure successes are strengthened, this "exposure works" schema may be expanded into a broader "that was then, this is now" formulation of improvement, which may take any of a number of forms: "I have changed, and I now know how to approach my fears differently, and that makes all the difference in the world"; "Now that I am more comfortable with my anxiety, every challenging situation is easier"; or "The things I have feared are just not as dangerous as I always assumed." Consistent with the documentation of sudden gains in therapy (where dramatic changes in symptoms occur from one session to the next), the early creation of ambivalent meaning to fear cues may lend itself to a more sudden resolution of these ambivalent meanings due to a subsequent clear test of the two expectancies in exposure, resulting in a sudden increase of learned safety.

In the chapters that follow, we discuss the possibility of formulating a hierarchy of fears for guiding treatment. One rationale for starting at a moderate level in this hierarchy is to have the opportunity to teach patients how to approach, attend to, and evaluate their exposures when anxiety, negative expectancies, and automatic avoidance responses are not overwhelmingly strong. Indeed, a subset of patients prefers that approach over immediately starting with cues that are higher on the hierarchy. Early, lower-level exposures give such patients a chance to learn how to approach exposures, that they can tolerate initial anxiety, and that exposure therapy can work. All of this learning is then usefully applied to subsequent higher-order exposures. For this reason, targeting the "low-hanging fruit" of easier-to-treat fears can be a useful clinical strategy (see Chapter 3). Initial successes provide the procedural and outcome memories to guide subsequent exposures for the patient.

2.4. Summary

In this chapter, we introduced a model of fears in terms of a network of learned associations that involve a complex set of memory elements that reflect cue associations across sensory modalities as well as language-based abstractions about these associations. These memories, when cued, determine the expectancies a person has about a feared situation or event. In exposure therapy, we are using therapeutic experience to change these expectancies of danger. If we provide inadequate or partial safety learning, the original fear memories and the new safety memories may sit side by side, each activated when the right cues are present. For full treatment, we want to target core fear memories, not just provide a special case of memories (e.g., "Giving a speech is terrifying, but giving a speech when my clinician is present is less so"). The process of changing fear-related expectancies relies on the salience, context specificity, and scope of the safety learning.

A core message of this chapter is that safety learning from exposure therapy is not a passive process; instead, it is the active learning of safety in response to fear cues. Accordingly, procedures that enhance the salience and breadth of the safety memories improve outcome. What the patient is thinking about and attending to before, during, and after exposure matters. In this chapter, we have drawn attention to the importance of

(1) Setting up active learning by clarifying expectancies for relevant fear cues.
(2) Actively testing these expectancies relative to well-defined exposure outcomes.
(3) Clear postexposure processing of what was (and was not) learned from the exposure.
(4) Rehearsal of this learning in the interval between sessions.

We also underscored the importance of generalizing safety learning across contexts, fading the use of safety cues/behaviors, and making sure that safety learning is not conditional.

In brief, during exposure therapy, you teach patients the difference between safety and danger (i.e., false alarms vs. true alarms), and help them replace experiences of perceived threat with their new experiences of safety. By planning exposure sessions that sequentially better match core cues for fear over time and better eliminate derailing contexts (safety cues) over time, you can provide their patients with more indelible memories of safety, leading to long-lasting benefits from exposure therapy.

3
General Approach

3.1. Principal Assumptions

Exposure therapy targets the formation of strong safety memories. These memories are aided by the active processing of the exposure practice. To develop a new (safety) memory that can effectively compete with the original fear memory,

(1) The patient and clinician must have a good understanding of the original fear memory (**planning for exposure therapy**).
(2) The new experiences provided by exposure therapy must accurately and unambiguously contradict the threat expectations driven by the original fear memories (**delivery of exposure therapy**).
(3) The new learning that takes place during exposure therapy sessions must cement in the memory or be transferred from short-term to long-term memory (**processing of exposure therapy**).

Aiming to provide you with a roadmap for the effective implementation of exposure therapy, this chapter describes the three stages—planning, delivery, and processing—and serves as the basis for chapters that follow. Specifically, we will describe the general approach in this chapter and then adapt it for the most common feared cues (emotions and related physical sensations, people, situations and objects, thoughts and images, traumatic memories) in the next set of chapters. We considered organizing the book by anxiety disorder rather than by fear cues. The reason we opted for the latter is that fear cues play a critical role in the *case formulation* that is at the heart of personalized exposure therapy. Indeed, we conceptualize anxiety, fear, and their disorders as a product of faulty threat appraisals triggered by one or more external (situations, objects, or people) and/or internal (emotions, physical sensations, thoughts, images, or traumatic memories) cues (see Figure 3.1).

Fear or panic is the product of a perception of danger that is around the corner or *immediate*, whereas anxiety emerges as a result of an appraisal of threat that occurs in a more distant *future*.

Placing the emphasis on specific fear cues also orients you toward a transdiagnostic approach to intervention. Rather than addressing comorbidity

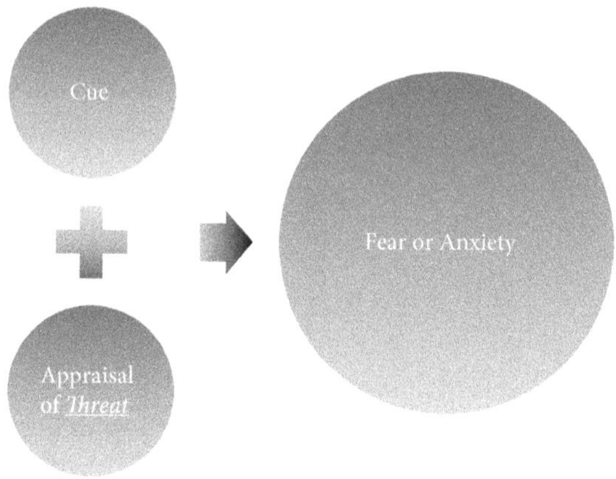

Figure 3.1 The main ingredients of fear/anxiety.

by treating the different disorders sequentially, the focus on assessing fear cues, the responses they elicit, and the core concerns that maintain this stimulus–response relationship encourages you to develop a more efficient treatment plan—one that centers on the core targets that explain the comorbidity. Consider Jorge, a 43-year-old male with a diagnosis of major depressive disorder, panic disorder, and social anxiety disorder. He would likely benefit from receiving three diagnostic-specific interventions offered in sequence, but it is more efficient to develop an intervention that targets the factor(s) that fuel(s) his emotions, in his case a concern of being perceived as incompetent (see Figure 3.2). The efficient and likely more potent treatment plan for Jorge is to intervene on the "phobia" of being perceived as incompetent.

As we discuss the planning stage, we help you fine-tune your assessment tactics during the initial phases of treatment—the aim here is to help you collect the information you need to develop a case formulation that will guide the selection of exposure exercises. Although guiding a patient in confronting their feared stimuli is simple in principle, the success of exposure therapy can greatly vary depending on your actions as you work with the patient through these exercises. We will discuss the dos and don'ts when delivering exposure therapy, highlighting common traps clinicians face and how to avoid them, and introducing in-session strategies that help you keep the patient on track. Lastly, fostering new memories of safety that can effectively compete with existing fear memories requires that we as clinicians ensure adequate processing of new information that is made available during the sessions. The section on the processing of exposure therapy in this chapter introduces you to a series of strategies that can be employed to cement the learning that is essential to the staying power of exposure therapy.

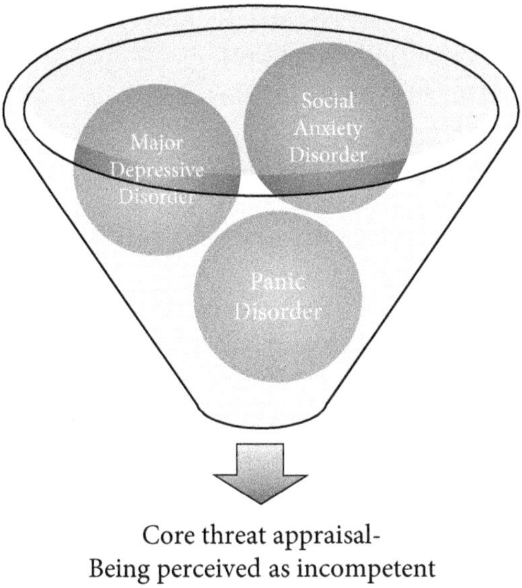

Figure 3.2 Transdiagnostic approach to exposure therapy.

3.2. Planning for Exposure Therapy

While acknowledging the limitations of psychological assessment and the fact that fully understanding a patient's emotional health problems may require multiple sessions over time, the following four steps are sufficient for developing an initial exposure therapy plan:

(1) phone call;
(2) questionnaire battery;
(3) intake interview; and
(4) self-monitoring.

3.2.1. Phone Call

We prefer to provide an initial framework for the first session by conducting a preliminary phone call. We understand that this preference may not be shared by all clinicians, and, as such, the following content can be shifted into the first face-to-face session. The objectives of this first contact interaction (by phone or in session) are to:

(1) Develop initial hypotheses about the core concerns maintaining the patient's anxiety and related problems.
(2) Orient the patient to exposure therapy.

Questions to keep in mind for this goal include:

- What cues does the patient fear, and what does he or she feel when cued (emotion and physiology)?
- What does he or she think when cued (specific catastrophic thoughts)?
- What does he or she do when cued (avoidance and safety behaviors)?

At the end of this interaction, the goal is to understand the patient's thoughts and framing of his or her fear so well that we can imagine reacting in exactly the same way if we had the same thoughts and actions in response to the fear cues. This is what we mean by identifying the core maintaining factors. Reaching this level of understanding improves our likelihood for good clinical outcome while building strong empathy and rapport. The patient feels well understood.

As we attend to these questions in the first interaction, we keep in mind that credibility and expectancy for change are important to therapeutic progress. Buy-in from the patient is more likely when he or she believes that we understand anxiety and fear and use effective methods to help treat these problems. A productive first interaction starts by setting an agenda stating the objectives and the activities. For example, for a preliminary phone call, this would include the following:

> I would like to talk with you for about 10 minutes before our first appointment. The goals are for me to learn more about what you want to focus on in therapy and to make sure that you come to our first session having an idea of what you can expect from working with me. So, we will spend a few minutes talking about what brings you to treatment, and then I will tell you briefly about how I go about therapy. How does that sound?"

The initial phone assessment has gone well if we leave with hypotheses about the core concerns driving the anxiety, as these will guide the development of a targeted follow-up assessment.

> So, Jorge, it is clear that you want to get rid of the panic attacks. Many people I see in my practice have panic attacks, and I know that the experience differs greatly from one person to the other. For us to develop a treatment plan that best meets *your* needs, I would just like to get a better idea of what panic attacks are like for you and what causes these to happen. Can you tell me what a panic

> attack feels like—the physical sensations? What sets them off—what are the triggers? And what goes through your mind when you experience panic—or the *uh oh* thoughts you have right before or during an attack? What exactly are you afraid may happen at the time (identify the specific perceived catastrophic outcome)?

Establishing a collaborator early on sets the stage for productive interactions during the therapeutic process. Patients, especially those new to therapy, often do not know what is expected from them and how they can best answer questions. By telling patients the aims of your questions, you help them organize their answers and encourage them to take on a role of "co-clinician"—someone who will work with you to understand the problem they want to address in therapy.

The information about the "cue–thought–feeling relation" shared during this initial conversation directs the assessment strategies in the subsequent three phases—the selection of questionnaire battery, the focus of the subsequent intake interview, and the targets for self-monitoring to be completed in the week following the intake interview.

> It seems that for you panic attacks are linked to social situations—the times when you are concerned that people take note of you and form a negative impression. One of the concerns driving your panic attacks is that people around you see you as incompetent, and especially when you have a panic attack. We are going to talk more about this when we meet next week, and to facilitate that meeting, I am going to ask you to complete some self-report measures before we meet. These measures will ask you some follow-up questions on feelings, thoughts, and actions—knowing about these and how they are connected is essential to the treatment that I prescribe. Let's talk a little bit more about exposure therapy. What do you know about it?"

It is reasonable that patients express some anxiety about the idea of confronting their fears and concern about its therapeutic effects. Indeed, patients often argue that exposure has "failed" them. Jorge, for example, could argue that he has continued to attend required work meetings and the occasional social gatherings, but despite this kind of "exposure," his anxiety and fears have persisted. On top of that, stories covering exposure therapy in the media have tended to highlight the challenge of exposure therapy—namely, tolerating distress. There is an opportunity in this initial contact to address these possible concerns. In addition to highlighting the strong evidence base for exposure therapy (see Chapter 10 for a listing of the facts), it is important that you emphasize the difference between confronting fears as they occur in daily life and exposure therapy. Consider sharing the following information:

(1) Exposure therapy has been studied in hundreds of clinical trials.
(2) The findings of these clinical trials support exposure therapy as a first-line intervention for the anxiety disorders.
  - Response rates are as high as 85%.
  - Attrition rates are around 20% and are comparable to other first-line interventions like medications.
(3) Exposure therapy is different from exposure as it occurs naturally in the real world. Proper exposure therapy is effective when it differs from naturalistic exposure in the following ways:
  - Exposure exercises will be *systematic* (using the exact same exposure stimuli selected by the patient and clinician—under the same conditions initially each time until fear declines), *deliberate* (the patient chooses and controls the exposure rather than the exposure controlling or surprising the patient), *prolonged* (staying with the exposure until the patient achieves goal), and *repeated* (doing an exposure once demonstrates courage but is not sufficient, and these repetitions should occur close together in time). These features are essential to learning to feel safe again.
  - Exposure practice ends with a review, ensuring that information made available during the exercise will be processed in a useful way.
(4) Exposure therapy is collaborative, such that the patient and clinician design the exercises together. The clinician serves as a coach, and the patient controls "the speed" of therapy

> I recognize that it is hard to imagine that confronting fears is an effective method for overcoming your problems with panic attacks. Why would you provoke fear when your goal is to get rid of it? It is difficult to come up with a satisfying answer when you also consider that you have been going to meetings—doing exposure—yet you continue to have panic attacks. So, let me try to provide more information that supports exposure therapy as the right approach. First, when we do exposure exercises in treatment, we plan them carefully together—we set specific goals that we can measure and then evaluate afterwards. Second, we do the exposure exercise not just once, but we do it repeatedly in a short time period. So, in that way, it is different from you speaking up at the monthly meeting in January and doing it again a year later. The way you described those natural exposures can be sensitizing or make you feel more anxious about the situation, whereas doing it more systematically, on purpose and repeatedly, actually results in a reduction in fear. We know this because exposure therapy has been studied like medications in clinical trials. Hundreds of trials have been carried out,

> showing response rates as high as 85%. Also, these studies show that, although it is hard work, most complete the full course of therapy, which is typically around 10 to 20 sessions. It is because of these successes that exposure therapy has been designated a first-line intervention for the anxiety disorders. So, how have I done in trying to convince you exposure therapy is a reasonable choice?"

One of the issues that we stress throughout the book as we review different procedures is that you make a habit of tracking success (see also Chapter 4). As you wrap up the interaction, review the goals and determine whether:

(1) You have identified possible core themes maintaining the presenting problem that you can further assess in the next stages.
(2) The patient has a sense of what they can expect from therapy with you.

> Thank you for spending a few minutes with me before we meet next week. I have some grasp of what sets off your panic attacks and why you keep having them. I am also glad that we had a chance to talk about exposure therapy, so that you have a better sense of what to expect when we get started. To help us be efficient when we meet next week, I am going to send you an orientation packet with some questionnaires. It would be great if you could bring that to the session.

3.2.2. Questionnaire Battery

The objectives of administering a questionnaire battery prior to the intake interview are to:

(1) Collect data to inform the case formulation.
(2) Orient the patient to a treatment that emphasizes the importance of assessment for evaluating progress and directing treatment decisions.

The new patient orientation packet includes the following documents: Informed consent, HIPAA privacy policy, HIPAA receipt, and background questionnaire (see www.oup.com/us/personalizedexposure for an example background questionnaire). The questionnaire battery that complements the new patient orientation packet cover three domains—emotion, appraisal, and action—central to the case formulation (see the chain in the shaded area in Figure 3.3).

Chapter 9 provides a list of validated assessment instruments and procedures organized by domain. Applying this to Jorge, the information gathered during

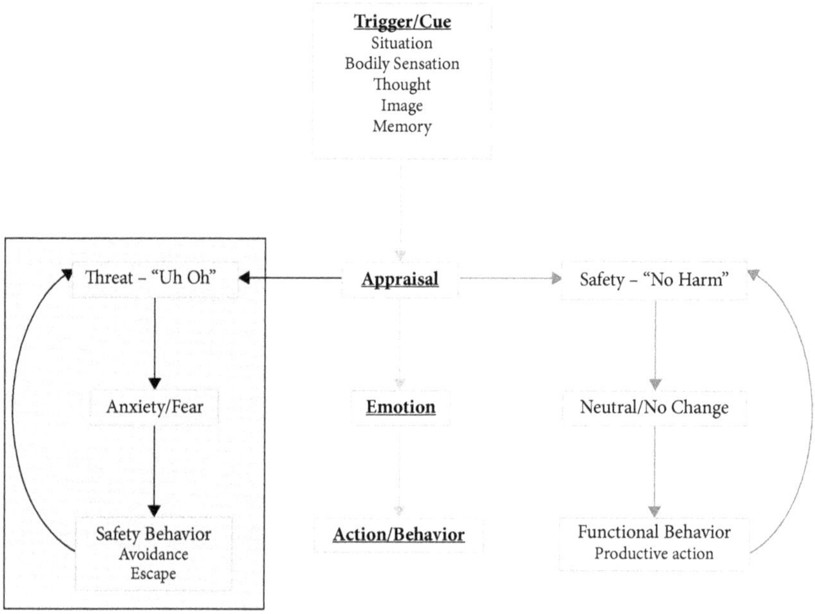

Figure 3.3 Maintaining factors in anxiety and related disorders.

the initial meeting pointed to problems with panic attacks (emotion), anxiety in social situations (emotion), and depressed mood (emotion), fueled, at least in part, by concerns about being perceived as incompetent (appraisal). Table 3.1 depicts a comprehensive assessment strategy that can be used to test these initial hypotheses.

3.2.3. Intake Interview

The main objectives of the intake interview are to:

(1) Establish diagnoses.
(2) Develop an initial case formulation.
(3) Develop an initial treatment plan.

The form that we use for the intake evaluation (see www.oup.com/us/personalizedexposure) maps onto the first two steps for exposure therapy planning—phone call and questionnaire battery. Much of the data collected during these first two phases (e.g., medical history, past psychiatric treatment history, family history, questionnaire scores) can be transcribed to the intake

Table 3.1 An Example Self-Report Battery

Instrument	Domain	Target
Panic Disorder Severity Scale (PDSS)	Symptoms	Panic disorder symptom severity
Liebowitz Social Anxiety Scale (LSAS)	Symptoms	Social anxiety disorder symptom severity
Patient Health Questionnaire (PHQ-9)	Symptoms	Depression symptom severity
Panic Appraisal Inventory-II (PAI-II)	Appraisal	Concerns about the consequences of panic
Anxiety Sensitivity Index (ASI)	Appraisal	Concerns about anxiety and related sensations
Appraisal of Social Concerns (ASC)	Appraisal	Concerns about social performance
Texas Safety Maneuver Scale (TSMS)	Action	Panic-related safety behaviors
Subtle Avoidance Frequency Examination (SAFE)	Action	Social anxiety-related safety behaviors

form prior to the session. This information can be briefly verified during the session, thus allowing more time to learn about the presenting problem.

> Thanks for completing the questionnaires and bringing these in, Jorge. This is very helpful for the session today. I will take a few minutes to review your responses and take some notes before we get started.

If you have access to a HIPAA-compliant online survey manager, you can request that the patient completes the information packet before the appointment, so that you can do the preparation work prior to the session. Either way, make a habit of acknowledging the completion of the "homework" assignment, making clear that you are using it to inform your sessions—or rewarding the patient for his or her effort. Not reviewing homework carefully dramatically decreases the likelihood of further homework completion. Highlighting that you appreciate the effort and that you will use the information likely enhances his or her motivation to complete subsequent assignments. We emphasize again that every session must start with setting an agenda. This sets the tone that this is an organized, focused intervention. It also has the positive side effect of reducing getting sidetracked by daily living and differentiating what we do relative to typical open-ended talk therapy.

> So, let's set the agenda for today's session. You'll get used to me setting the agenda at the beginning of each session—it's a way to help make sure that we make progress. My goal is for you to leave today with an idea of what treatment is going to be like. To develop a treatment plan, I would like to learn more about the panic attacks and feelings of anxiety and depression that you described during our brief phone call last week. It's also important that we talk about some other issues, such as your physical health and use of substances, as well as other possible stressors, because we know that these can affect your emotional health. I will be completing this evaluation form, and as you can see, I have already filled out some sections based on your responses on the questionnaires. We will start by reviewing these sections briefly, making sure that I have interpreted your responses correctly but then spend most the time talking about what brings on panic attacks, feelings of anxiety and depression for you, and how you respond to these feelings. I will leave some time at the end to give you some impressions, which includes diagnoses as well as an initial treatment plan. We will finish the session developing a brief exercise that you can complete before our first treatment session. Before we get started with this though, I would like to tell you a bit more about myself, giving you a chance to ask some questions that you may have about me. Do you have anything else that you would like to add to the agenda?"

3.2.4. Initial Case Formulation

When discussing the presenting problem, we collect information about the onset, course, and severity. To further inform the *case formulation*, we want to better understand *cue-appraisal-emotion-action* relation (see Figure 3.4). Specifically, using questionnaire data (see Chapter 9) as a guide, your interview should be focused on gathering information about the following:

(1) *Cues.* What is at the onset of the shift in affect? Cues can be internal (thoughts, images, bodily sensations, memories) or external (situations, people).
(2) *Thoughts.* What is the *uh oh* thought, and what is the theme (or are the themes) that drive(s) this *uh oh* thought? The vulnerability or danger

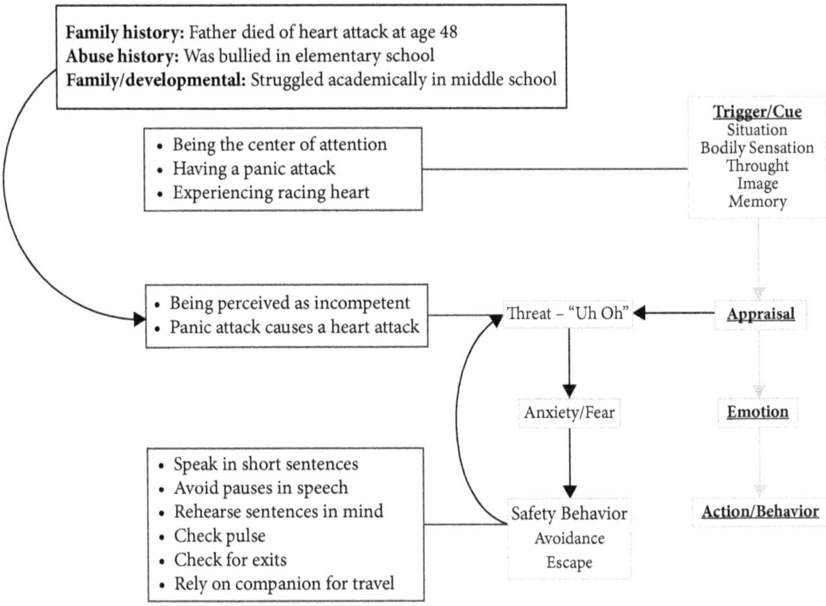

Figure 3.4 An example initial case formulation.

themes that drive anxiety can be present (fear, panic) or future (anxiety, worry) oriented and can include "catastrophes" across different domains (e.g., physical health, mental health, work/school, relationships, functioning).

(3) *Feelings.* What emotions and bodily sensations occur in response to these cues (fear, heart racing)?

(4) *Actions.* What does the patient do (safety behaviors) to manage the fear/ anxiety (e.g., escape, avoidance, substance use, reassurance seeking)?

We like bringing questionnaire data to the session, as it underscores to the patient that we value their homework completion, and it can help direct the patient to talk about themes that are central to the maintenance of their anxiety problems.

> I have highlighted a few responses on the questionnaires that asked you about how you cope with anxiety in social situations and panic attacks. You report that you often speak in short sentences, you often avoid pauses in your speech, and you always rehearse sentences in mind. We refer to these habits as safety behaviors—these are actions that enhance your sense of safety. It makes sense to me that you have developed these habits or crutches—you said you are

> concerned about being perceived as incompetent and thus you try to optimize the chances of a good performance, right?

This is a reminder that, because they serve a specific function, behaviors can provide great insight into the core concerns driving anxiety and panic. A careful assessment of safety behaviors can therefore be very helpful in performing differential diagnosis and developing or tweaking the case formulation.

> You also report always checking for exits; usually check your pulse, breathing, blood pressure; and you always rely on a companion for travel to manage your panic. These safety behaviors suggest that, in addition to being the center of attention, you are also concerned about other possible consequences of panic attacks. Your responses to some other items make it clear that you are also afraid that a panic attack may cause a heart attack. Is that the concern that drives the use of those safety behaviors?

Sections in the interview on current stressors, medical history, medication history, and substance use further aid differential diagnosis—that is, rule out conditions that may explain the presenting problem(s)—whereas other sections (e.g., treatment history, family history, abuse history, family/developmental) can help you fine-tune the case formulation, providing you with a context for understanding the origins of certain threat appraisals (see Figure 3.4).

The questionnaire responses and the interview make it clear that Jorge meets diagnostic criteria for social anxiety disorder (fueled by concerns about being perceived as incompetent) and panic disorder (fueled by concerns about the physical consequences of panic attacks). Like is true for many patients, these disorders have caused impairments in many domains in his life, resulting in the symptoms consistent with major depressive disorder. Note again that, although it's important to document diagnoses, the case formulation-oriented approach identifies the maintaining processes as opposed to the disorder(s) as main targets for intervention, predicting that, in Jorge's case, intervening on "being perceived as incompetent" and "panic causes physical harm" will be required to achieve his treatment goals.

You wrap up the session by providing your patient with feedback—your initial impressions (e.g., diagnoses, case formulation)—and link this to the initial treatment plan and your follow-up assessment.

> Before we end today's session, I want to give you my impressions, making sure I have interpreted what you have said correctly, and then I can tell you more about what I believe is a reasonable treatment plan.

> The experiences you describe are consistent with what we see in panic disorder, social anxiety disorder, and major depressive disorder. I know that sounds like a lot, but these three diagnoses are closely linked and often go together. Panic disorder and social anxiety disorder are similar in that they are both characterized by anxiety/panic and avoidance but they are different in terms of the content of the worry. Panic disorder is fueled by a fear of panic attacks—or the fear of fear—while social anxiety disorder is fueled by a fear of rejection. Given the impact of panic and anxiety on your social and work life, it's not surprising that you have also developed depression. So, I expect that if we treat panic and social anxiety disorder, you will also see your depression lifted.
>
> As you can see in the diagram, we can knock out panic and social anxiety disorder if we target the *uh oh* thoughts and safety behaviors. That brings us back to exposure therapy. What do you remember from our phone conversation?"

Much of the first treatment session will be devoted to discussing the exposure therapy rationale and procedures, so the conversation at the end of this session can be brief. The main objective here is to ensure that the patient has a general sense of exposure therapy, recognizes that it's effective, and is open to trying it.

> You have a good sense of what exposure therapy is going to be like. When we meet next week, we will talk more about how we apply exposure therapy to target your fears. Assessment will be a key component to our work together. I am going to be asking you to complete questionnaires every week so that I can see whether we are on track or whether we need to change course. For this upcoming week, I am going to ask you to complete a daily record of your anxiety, panic and mood.

In this section, we presented the "best case scenario" for an intake assessment in the office with all of our recourses. We recognize that some settings only permit brief "on the fly" assessments (e.g., consultation/liaison). In those settings, the format presented for the initial phone call can be complemented by a brief assessment of MAPS—mood, anxiety, psychosis, and substance use/suicide.

3.2.5. Self-Monitoring

The objectives of self-monitoring are to:

(1) Test hypotheses about the core concerns maintaining the anxiety and related problems, or the validity of the initial case formulation.

(2) Reinforce the importance of assessment for evaluating progress and directing treatment decisions.

Assigning homework after the intake evaluation reinforces the message that the patient is an active participant or collaborator in treatment. The "work" that he or she does between sessions facilitates treatment progress and provides feedback regarding the case formulation as well as the effects of the intervention strategies. Recognizing that any assignment adds to the existing workload and this can be perceived as a burden, the homework prescription is a collaboration between you and the patient, balancing "needs" with feasibility. We recommend that clinicians complete the initial monitoring form as well understand the assignment and burden. In fact, as a general rule we state, "Never ask a patient to do anything you have not done yourself first." A closely related theme is that we recommend you never assign homework that you have not first practiced in session with the patient. Thus, for self-monitoring, it can be helpful to not only go over the form but to fill one out together. We give the instruction to fill one out with us covering the "worst" previous episode as an example.

> Our last item on today's agenda is to develop a homework exercise that you can complete before our first therapy session. Hardly anyone that I know likes the term *homework*, but home practice is crucial to getting better for any type of course you take—and the research supports that. Think about it like you're training for a race, and I am your running coach. We meet weekly to run a few miles together, which is helpful, but we both know that if you also run on your own you are going to have a better race. So, we will finish all our sessions from now on designing some specific exercises that can help reinforce the learning that takes place in the session. For the next week, I believe it would be useful if you kept a daily record of your thoughts, actions, and feelings. Our conversation today has helped us identify some possible themes that drive your emotions, and I think it would be good to see whether they actually play out that way or whether there are perhaps themes that we have overlooked. I put together a simple form (see Box 3.1) that you can complete each time you experience a panic attack or a noticeable increase in anxiety. In the event you experience no such anxiety over the next week, we would still like you to fill out the form using other previous example episodes to go over next week. Let's review it together to see whether this makes sense or needs any updating.

Box 3.1 An Example Self-Monitoring Form

Please complete this after you experience a panic attack or (increase in) anxiety.

- Panic/Anxiety:
  - Intensity (0–100):
- Day:
- Time:
- Situation:
- Tigger/Cue:
  - Situation:
  - Bodily sensation:
  - Thought:
  - Image:
- "Uh oh" thought:
- Safety behavior(s):

3.3. Delivery of Exposure Therapy

3.3.1. Socialization to the Exposure Therapy Model

In the next session, you transition from preparing for exposure therapy to delivering exposure therapy. You process the latest assessment data that include the self-monitoring homework assignment as well as the scores on the measures the patient completed prior to the session (see assessment schedule for Jorge in Table 3.2) and aim to have developed a first exposure exercise by the end of the session.

> Today, we are getting started with treatment. I would like to begin with a review of the homework and then spend the rest of the time working on developing an initial exposure exercise. Do you have anything else you want to add to the agenda?

Homework review in the first session serves the function of reinforcing the importance of "working" between sessions—signaling to the patient that these contributions pay off. The review of the self-monitoring will center around verifying the initial case formulation by reviewing whether the hypothesized

Table 3.2 An Example Assessment Schedule

Instrument	Frequency
Panic Disorder Severity Scale (PDSS)	Weekly
Liebowitz Social Anxiety Scale (LSAS)	Weekly
Patient Health Questionnaire (PHQ-9)	Bi-weekly
Panic Appraisal Inventory-II (PAI-II)	Weekly
Anxiety Sensitivity Index (ASI)	Every three weeks
Appraisal of Social Concerns (ASC)	Every three weeks
Texas Safety Maneuver Scale (TSMS)	Every three weeks
Subtle Avoidance Frequency Examination (SAFE)	Every three weeks

maintaining factors—threat appraisals and safety behaviors—are actually operating in the anxiety/panic episodes experienced during the week. It's possible that the self-monitoring reveals actions or cognitive themes that are different from those discussed during the assessment phase, which prompts you to update your case formulation and corresponding treatment targets/plan. For example, if Jorge's self-monitoring form shows that he panicked when he felt dizzy because he predicted he was going to lose control, adding loss of control as a maintaining factor may be implicated (see Chapters 5–7 for example diagrams for case formulations). This would impact your treatment planning to include exposure practice that allows Jorge to learn that panic does not lead to loss of control (even if it feels like it).

The weekly administration of questionnaires helps you determine whether you are on track, not only in terms of meeting the patient's goals (see Chapter 9 for cut-offs for remission) but also with respect to assessing whether you are successful in engaging the targets responsible for symptom improvement. Sharing the scores (and their interpretation) as well the change in scores with the patient is an important part of the session, because clinicians see better outcomes with patients when they get into a habit of providing feedback. Patients are particularly interested to see their progress documented in this way. Think about weight loss. Physical trainers will often have clients weigh in weekly. Although the client already has a sense of how their clothes fit, what their scale says at home, how their diet and exercise regimens or progressing, they are still highly engaged in finding out their weight and body composition results with the trainer each week. This is no less true with psychological measures in exposure therapy work.

Much of the work completed in the previous phases helps provide the patient a context for interpreting the new learning that takes place during exposure practice. We cannot emphasize enough how important it is for a patient to understand the aims and procedures of exposure—a lack of symptom improvement over the course of exposure sessions can often be attributed to poor socialization to the exposure therapy model. Hence, before starting the exposure exercises, you devote the time and sessions needed to ensure that you and the patient approach the therapy sessions with the same goal (i.e., safety learning) and, importantly, you continue to assess patients on this variable (i.e., socialization to exposure therapy) as you move through treatment (for tracking success, see Chapter 4).

> As we start our treatment sessions, you'll find that I will often ask you about what you are getting out of the sessions—questions like, what did you take away from that exercise? And what about that is useful to you? These questions make clear that this treatment focuses on new learning, or building new memories of safety that compete with the old memory of danger, and that building these new memories is responsible for helping you achieve your goal to feel better. I've found that it's easier for patients to approach the sessions as a time to focus on learning if they have a good understanding of what keeps their anxiety going and how exposure therapy can help knock it out. We have talked about this over the past few meetings, but I wondered what has stuck from that for you?

The checklist presented in Box 3.2 may be useful as you determine whether the patient has been sufficiently socialized to exposure therapy.

You use the materials presented in Chapter 10 if you find that the patient requires additional education before starting exposure therapy. When reviewing the exposure rationale and procedures, acknowledge the seemingly opposing goals of the *therapy process*—inducing anxiety (and changing the response to develop memories of safety)—and *therapy outcome*—reducing anxiety.

> Okay, I want to spend a bit more time talking about the therapy rationale and procedures. It's got to be a bit strange for you that this therapy involves exercises that make you anxious when you come to me with the goal to feel less anxious. I'll be honest, I would also prefer a method that doesn't require that kind of effort. So why confront fears? What are the benefits of bringing on fear on purpose? Let's start by reviewing what happens when you don't confront fears and instead avoid or escape using the safety behaviors we have discussed. I am going to draw this on the whiteboard for you.

Box 3.2 Checklist for Assessing Socialization to Exposure Therapy

Patient recognizes

- ☐ That threat appraisals fuel the cue–anxiety/panic relation.
- ☐ That an appraisal of immediate threat produces panic whereas an appraisal of future threat produces anxiety.
- ☐ That anxiety and panic serve a protective function.
- ☐ That avoidance or escape are natural responses to anxiety/panic.
- ☐ The difference between a true an false alarm.
- ☐ That safety behaviors in response to a false alarm maintain the cue–threat appraisal-anxiety/panic relation.

Patient understands

- ☐ That exposure exercises are designed to reestablish a sense of safety around the feared cues.
- ☐ That exposure therapy differs from exposure in real life (deliberate, systematic, prolonged, repeated).
- ☐ That preventing safety behavior use during exposure is critical to developing the new memory of safety.
- ☐ That exposure exercises are successful when he or she does not "fight" the anxiety but instead learns to "relax" with/do nothing about it.
- ☐ That the design of exposure exercises will be done collaboratively.

As you can see here (see Figure 3.5), when you enter a feared situation, like a meeting, your fear increases until you decide to use a safety behavior. That's the beauty of safety behaviors—they are effective; they help you manage or reduce your fear. And, that's exactly why you continue to use them. Now, let me add some additional lines to this figure to show you why safety behaviors are problematic.

This graph (see Figure 3.6) showing the same curves illustrates the cycle that defines an anxiety disorder. You have learned to respond to fear by using your safety behaviors because they deliver every time. The problem, though, is that your fears and anxieties have persisted. Your habit has not helped you get rid of anxiety, but, in fact, as I will show you next, helped maintain it instead.

I've drawn next to this figure a revised curve (see Figure 3.7) that tells you what happens with fear when you change your habit—when you resist

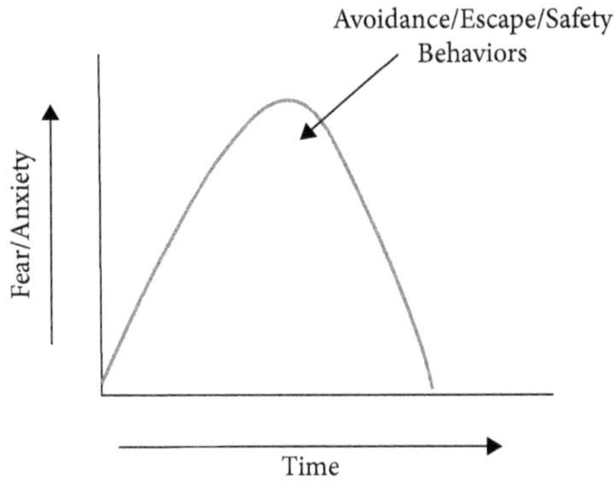

Figure 3.5 Rewarding properties of avoidance/escape.

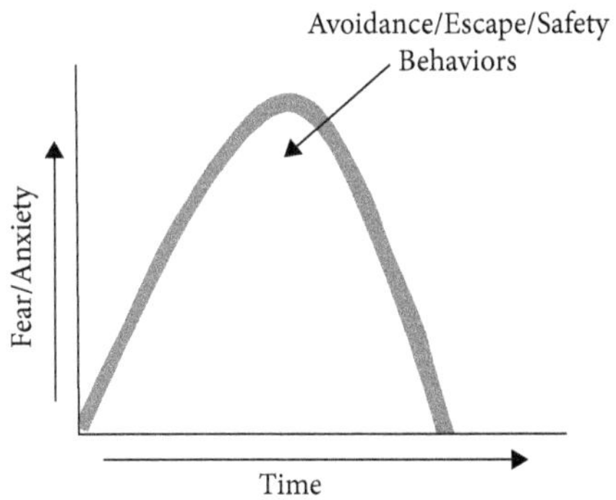

Figure 3.6 The anxiety disorder cycle.

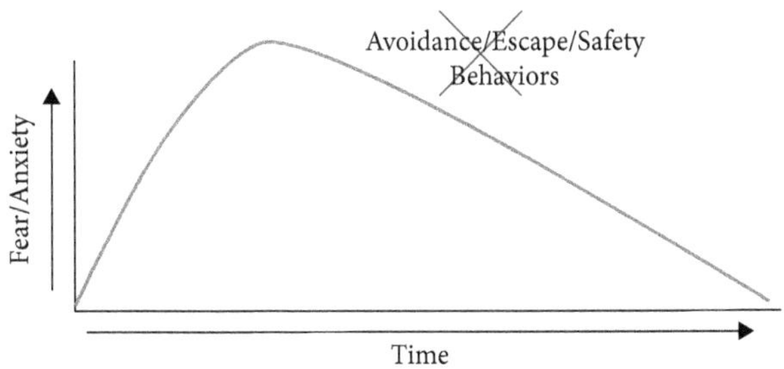

Figure 3.7 Removing safety behaviors.

engaging in safety behaviors. You can see that when you decide to respond to fear by *doing nothing*—just letting it be—the fear also goes down. Following the peak in symptoms that is guided by your sympathetic nervous system, your parasympathetic nervous system kicks in, which results in a returning of these symptoms to baseline. On top of that, and this is important, removing the safety behaviors allows you to see that you are having a false alarm—what you are afraid would happen does not happen after all. As in, experiencing very high fear or a panic attack, although uncomfortable, will not cause physical harm.

I'll admit that this curve seems less appealing than the one resulting from the use of safety behaviors. Take a look at this next figure (see Figure 3.8). It demonstrates the effects of exposure therapy. With repeated exposure exercises, your peak fear gets lower and your return to baseline becomes faster. The term for this process is *fear extinction*—it is something that observed across species. This graph emphasizes the importance of repetition. This is why exposure therapy is different from just attending a meeting once in a while. That is, exposure therapy involves the planning of confronting a feared situation on purpose and then do it over and over again so that you simply get bored with it.

Let me add to this or make clear that *letting the fear be* as I just indicated is a really important piece to effective exposure therapy. Remember, your habit is to fight fear—trying to push it away. In exposure therapy, we bring on fear on purpose to learn to change this habit and thus much of the work in the session will be focused on making sure that all your actions—and these can be subtle—clearly signal to your brain that you're safe. In essence, I am going to help you *act* normal even though you don't feel normal. We know that once you become consistent with your actions, your thoughts and feelings will follow. It's like a train—the engine or your actions leave the station well before the last cars or your thoughts and feelings start moving.

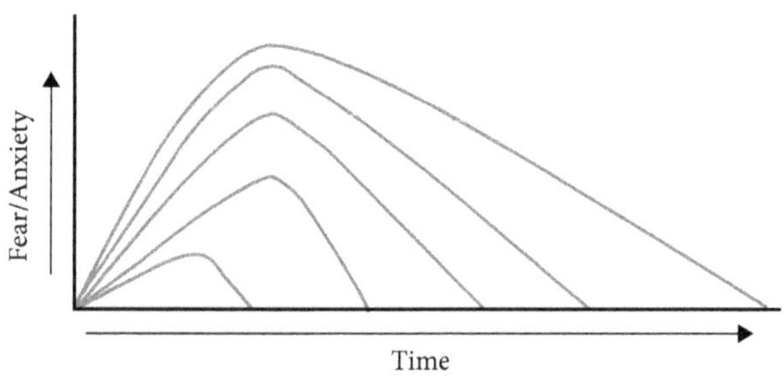

Figure 3.8 Fear extinction with exposure therapy.

3.3.2. Developing the Exposure Exercise

Before settling on the specific feared cue(s) and the parameters of the first exposure exercise, you will introduce the Subjective Units of Distress (SUDs) scale (see Figure 3.9). This introduction involves drawing the scale on the whiteboard (and/or providing a handout), reviewing the anchors with the patient, and discussing examples of situations for each of the major anchors (e.g., "Can you give me an example of a recent social situation where you felt hyped up but could cope or experienced a SUDs level of 25?").

In general, we aim to generate initial exposure scenarios that produces an initial SUDs level of 60 to 70. We believe that SUDs at that level indicate that patients have matched the cues of the exposure exercise with the cues of their core fears, which provides a sound basis for learning. And, for the learning to be relevant or therapeutic, the information yielded by the exposure exercise has to contradict the expectations that are driven by the fear memories. Effective contradiction depends on matching the content of relevant fear cues ("It will be really bad under X conditions") with similar safety outcomes ("It wasn't as bad as I expected under X conditions"). Your case formulation guides you in setting the "personalized" safety learning targets for the exposure session. For Jorge, for example, there are several desired take-home messages including but not limited to:

- I experienced high levels of fear but I didn't have a heart attack.
- I worried that I was going to appear anxious, but I ended coming across OK.
- I made social errors, but it ended up not mattering (no social cost).
- I achieved my goals, despite being anxious.

One important condition for effective exposure exercises is that the learning occurs without the presence of safety behaviors. Safety behaviors negatively reinforce anxiety by causing it to come back more often and teaching the patient that the only reason he or she was able to get through the exposure is because of the safety behavior, not because the exposure exercise wasn't dangerous.

In summary, you aim to induce initial fear by selecting relevant cues and then to help the patient "act" normal, allowing him or her to learn that the situation is much safer than expected. Thus, your goal is to make sure the exposure is

SUDS–Distress, Anxiety, or Emotional Discomfort

0	5	10	15	20	25	30	35	40	45	50	55	60	65	70	75	80	85	90	95	100
No anxiety, calm, relaxed					Mild anxiety, alert, able to cope					Moderate anxiety, some trouble concentrating					Severe anxiety, thoughts of leaving					Very severe anxiety, extreme fear

Figure 3.9 Subjective Units of Distress Scale.

relevant (initial SUDs in the target range of 60–70) and thereafter to have the patient learn contradictory information in the presence of these cues. We expect that the patient's SUDs will drop as this information is learned (see Figure 3.8), though, in some cases, the integration of the contradictory information may not occur until the patient completes the postexposure reflection on his or her exposure. For those patients, the decline in SUDs during the exposure exercise as seen in Figures 3.7 and 3.8 occurs in subsequent repetitions of the exercise when he or she has also learned to relinquish control—when he or she fully and consistently embraces the fear and allows it to run its course.

> Now that you are familiar with the SUDs scale, we can develop a first exposure exercise. We are going to do this together, but let me review the two key components of an effective exercise, so that you can keep those in mind as we plan this. First, we want to select a situation or cue that generates SUDs of around 60 or 70. At that level, we know that you are concerned about harm in some way and have a strong desire to escape. Therefore, it creates a great opportunity for learning—allowing you to practice relaxing with the fear to learn that you are safe. Second, we want to complete the exercise without relying on crutches or safety behaviors. Our goal is to demonstrate that safety around this cue is clear-cut or unconditional. Using crutches gets in the way of seeing that your threat predictions are unfounded regardless of what you do in the situation.
>
> Let's take a look at this planning sheet (see Box 3.3). As you can see, I have already completed several of the sections based on your responses on the questionnaires you completed before the session today. These are ideas that I know can make for a great exercise. I am curious about your thoughts about this though—let's get your input and develop the specifics of this first exposure exercise."

It's easy to fall into the trap of underdosing the exposure exercise. Patients are nervous about confronting feared cues, have a tendency to avoid, and often are unsure that they can persist in a situation that produces high fear levels. One way to respond to this is by developing a first task that the patient sees as easily manageable—easing into it. Although tempting and certainly reflecting caring for the patient, doing so can greatly undermine the efficacy and efficiency of therapy. The risk we run by promoting avoidance is that we inadvertently communicate that we perceive the procedures as risky potentially causing harm to the patient. Because we are targeting false alarms and perceive the patient's avoidance maneuvers as a maladaptive habit—patients have "temporarily" adopted safety behaviors (or moved away from their normal routine) simply to manage their (unfounded) fears—it is critical that we signal confidence early on. When we as clinicians are directive in this early phase, proposing an exercise that requires

Box 3.3 An Example Exposure Planning Worksheet

Patient: *Jorge* **Date:** *1-13-2017*

Target threat appraisals (use response on the *ASC* and *PAI-2*):
Feared outcome: *being perceived as incompetent* Rating: *80%*
Feared outcome: *having a heart attack* Rating: *25%*
Feared outcome: Rating:
Feared outcome: Rating:

Goals
Induce initial SUDs level of 60–70 and disconfirm the feared outcomes.

Situation/Cue
- ❑ Social interaction: *meeting a stranger*
- ❑ Bodily sensation(s): *racing heart*
- ❑ Social performance: *giving a speech*
- ❑ Other cue(s):

Manipulations to Achieve Match to Fear Cues
- ❑ Interaction/performance topic:
- ❑ Duration (specify minutes): minutes
- ❑ Fade other safety cues/behavior (s) (use response on ***the SAFE and TSMQ***): List targeted safety cue/behaviors: *check pulse, rehearse sentences in mind, speak in short sentences, avoid pauses in speech*
- ❑ Induction of interoceptive sensations (list): *running in place*
- ❑ Social errors/mishaps (specify): *ums and ahs, drawing a blank, saying something that's incorrect*
- ❑ Feedback: *ask other for ratings of performance*

Set specific and achievable behavioral goal (based on goals and manipulations):
Complete 45-second trials of stair climbing, resisting the urge to stop.

Notes: ASC = Appraisal of Social Concerns scale; PAI-2 = Panic Appraisal Inventory-2; SAFE = Subtle Avoidance Frequency Examination; TSMQ = Texas Safety Maneuvers Questionnaire.

considerable courage, we model confidence and communicate our belief that (a) exposure is effective and (b) the patient *is* strong even though he or she may not *feel* strong. So, the default is to start by generating the ideal scenario—one that pushes the envelope, maximizing the opportunity to send a message of safety. Note that in Box 3.3, in addition to targeting the fading of the various safety behaviors during the exercise, pushing the envelope involves asking the patient to engage in antagonistic actions—behaviors that are the direct opposite of the automated safety maneuvers. By asking Jorge to intentionally make errors during a social interaction or performance (i.e., showing the signs he associates with incompetence), he avoids leaving the sessions with some of the common "what ifs" that can weaken the learning of any exposure exercise. When Jorge acts like he is not concerned about being perceived as incompetent, he can begin to learn that most social encounters carry minimal significance even if he comes across as inept.

3.3.3. Deviating from the Default

Ideally, we start with an exercise that yields unambiguous evidence of safety. Indeed, pushing the envelope from the beginning has been shown to be effective and has the benefit of speeding up treatment for patients who are willing and able to go at that pace. This default approach to exposure practice also helps you as you strive to be consistent in terms of modeling the view of an anxiety disorder and the confidence in exposure therapy—that is, "I know this is very difficult, but we know these are false alarms, and I am confident that with effort and practice you can turn off these alarms." Exposure therapy is a collaborative effort, however, and thus the patient remains in control in terms of deciding about completing any exposure exercise. So, what to do when, despite coaching, a patient passes up on carrying out the prescribed exercise because they believe it is too difficult? How to deviate from the default depends on what drives the patient's reluctance. We describe two common underlying themes here and provide some guidance on how to alter the prescription to address these.

3.3.3.1. The "I Don't Buy This" Patient

Especially after what we believe was a productive intake process and first session, it's easy to forget how challenging it is for some patients to conceive of responding differently to their experience of anxiety. Instead of talking about intervening involving "changing the relation with fear from avoidance to approach," our patients tend to have discussions with their friends and loved ones about coping: "What can I do to get rid of this feeling or avoid it altogether?" So, it cannot be surprising when the patient simply declines to engage in a courageous act because he or she doesn't believe it will work. This patient can indicate that rationale is sensible, yet is unconvinced it works for him or her. For this patient, the initial focus of exposure exercises may not center on violating specific harm expectancies per se (i.e., the default), but instead on the factor that can facilitate this goal, namely, experiencing that his or her system works like that of any other person: His or her fear declines with repeated exposure exercises. It's one thing to hear a good story; it's another thing to see it for yourself. So, for this reluctant patient, the worksheet may be modified as illustrated in Box 3.4.

> Jorge, I am like you in that I have to see things before I believe it. I understand that it can seem to be too good to be true that simply getting yourself in the

Box 3.4 Exposure Planning Worksheet Targeting Anxiety Sensitivity

Patient: *Jorge* **Date:** *1-13-2017*

Target threat appraisals (use response on the *ASC* and *PAI-2*):

Feared outcome: Rating:

Feared outcome: *having a heart attack* Rating: 25%

Feared outcome: Rating:

Feared outcome: Rating:

Goals

Induce initial SUDs level of 40 and demonstrate that SUDs will decrease with repetition.

Situation/Cue

- ❑ Social interaction:
- ❑ Social performance:
- ❑ Bodily sensation(s): Racing heart
- ❑ Other cue(s):

Manipulations to Achieve Match to Fear Cues

- ❑ Interaction/performance topic:
- ❑ Duration (specify minutes):
- ❑ Fade other safety cues/behavior (s) (use response on the *SAFE* and *TSMQ*):
  List targeted safety cue/behaviors: *check pulse*
- ❑ Induction of interoceptive sensations (list): *running in place*
- ❑ Social errors/mishaps (specify):
- ❑ Feedback:

Set specific and achievable behavioral goal (based on goals and manipulations above):

Complete 45-second trials of stair climbing, resisting the urge to stop.

Notes: ASC = Appraisal of Social Concerns scale; PAI-2 = Panic Appraisal Inventory-2; SAFE = Subtle Avoidance Frequency Examination; TSMQ = Texas Safety Maneuvers Questionnaire.

feared situation over and over again will help you get over the fear. Why don't we make that the goal of the session today—having you leave seeing that your system is no different? Once you see that exposure works, I think you'll be ready to increase the intensity.

I am thinking we start with stair climbing here in the building. I know that 45 seconds going up without stopping will cause your heart to race. Based on what you said earlier, I figured that an exercise like that would produce some fear, like around a 40. Does that seem right? Notice that I am proposing eight uninterrupted reps and no checking of pulse. What do you think a set of exercises like that would yield?

3.3.3.2. The "Unwilling" Patient

We ask patients to engage in courageous acts. Many patients are able to effectively leverage previous experiences that involved successfully persisting in an effort that was hard emotionally or physically. It can be helpful, for example, to ask a patient who ran track in high school to recount handling successfully difficult practice sessions and describe the parallel with exposure therapy prior to beginning exposure exercises. Similarly, most patients will remember leaving home for the first time, resisting escape and just letting the emotions run their course. There are also patients, on the other hand, who will say that they always sidestep intense feelings and cannot point to emotionally intense experiences in which they persevered. The lack of experiences with satisfactorily managing intense emotions can cause patients to be cautious and can explain why they may not be willing to start an exposure exercise that produces SUDs levels of around 60 to 70. The key to success of exposure therapy with these patients is to target their emotional sensitivity and intolerance. Doing this early in the therapy can facilitate engagement in exposure therapy, allowing the patient to get the full benefits.

When unwillingness is driven by concerns about harmful (physical, emotional, or social) consequences of anxiety and related bodily sensations—also called anxiety sensitivity (see Chapter 9 for strategies to assess anxiety sensitivity)—it makes most sense to center initial exposure exercises on feared benign bodily sensations. Chapter 5 focuses on targeting the fears of emotions and related physical sensations and describes the procedures for exposure to bodily sensations or interoceptive exposure in detail. In short, interoceptive exposure involves completing actions that produce the feared bodily sensations without relying on safety behaviors. For Jorge, it is possible that his concerns about a panic attack causing a heart attack would get in the way of fully engaging in the public speaking exposure exercises targeting his fears of negative evaluation. Following a set of running exercises, which can illustrate that racing heart is indeed benign, Jorge would benefit from other panicogenic exercises like voluntary hyperventilation or inhalation of carbon dioxide-enriched air aimed at reducing emotional sensitivity by providing clear evidence that panic attacks are harmless. Allowing

Jorge to focus on learning to feel safe when he is the center of attention *after* he knows that a panic attack is not going to get him will make this exposure exercise more productive.

When a patient is unwilling because he or she simply cannot imagine being able to tolerate intense emotions—also called distress intolerance (see Chapter 9 for strategies to assess distress intolerance and Chapter 5 for strategies to treat it)—initial therapeutic exercises should be geared toward helping patients achieve success persisting while being upset. This can be most easily accomplished within the context of the targeted exposure exercises. Instead of starting at a SUDs of 60 to 70, you work with the patient to design an exercise that activates fear but at a level that would offer a moderate (as opposed to an overwhelming) challenge for resisting escape. In negotiating with the patient, it is important to keep in mind the goal of this exercise (i.e., decreasing distress intolerance) and the possibility of falling into the trap of rewarding the positive qualities of avoidance.

> As I said when we first talked on the phone, therapy is about working together. I act as your coach, pushing you to do things that are hard that help you achieve your goal of knocking out your fears. But, obviously, I adapt when you're signaling that I am maybe pushing too hard. Trust me, you're not the first person bringing this up. It is not uncommon that when discussing this first exercise, people will say that they are not certain that they can complete it—that it's too intense. So, before we head in that direction, I would like to suggest that we first work together getting you to see that you *can* tolerate emotions, even though you *feel* like you can't. I believe that when you build more confidence around this, you will be in a better position to push harder in the exposure exercises.
>
> I'll admit that taking this slight detour comes with one challenge for me. I've been telling you that avoidance and safety behaviors get in the way of overcoming an anxiety disorder. As we plan on making some changes to exposure practice, it's easy to choose to move away from the goal to get rid of these. It's a slippery slope, and I want us to be aware of that. So, when modifying the exercise, I want to make sure that we make the goal persistence or completion—in other words, we focus on preventing your habit of escaping negative feelings. In doing so, we can initially allow some safety behaviors to ensure that the fear is not too high, but as your confidence builds, we will start fading these so that you can also see that avoidance is not required for you to be effective. I have revised the planning worksheet (see Box 3.5)—take a look and see what you think"

3.3.4. Systematic, Deliberate, Prolonged, and Repeated

Exposure therapy is only different from exposure to feared situations as they occur naturally (e.g., the occasional presentation at work, experimenting with cannabis while visiting a friend over the summer, the flight to attend the annual family reunion) and only effective when we prescribe it as an exercise for safety learning. Exposure is therapeutic when it is:

(1) *Systematic*—or involves a specific program aimed at helping patients re-establish a sense of safety around feared cues. The program involves careful planning and a collaboration between clinician and patient and is guided by the principles of safety learning.
(2) *Deliberate*—or when the patient determines the time and circumstances of his or her exposure practice. This is the opposite from the nontherapeutic spontaneous exposures he or she knows from his or her daily life, which are sensitizing. The clinician acts merely as a coach, allowing the patient to gain a sense of agency in his or her improvement.
(3) *Prolonged*—or when the completion of a goal (e.g., completing a flight, recounting the complete memory) instead of the drive to escape determines the end of an exposure exercise. Relating differently to a false alarm and appreciating it as such requires that the patient takes away the significance that escape places on the experience of false alarms.
(4) *Repeated*—or when the clinician and patient prioritize repetitions in the session and outside the session. Patients learn that safety is unambiguous and unconditional only when they do the exercise over and over again, first with the clinician and then outside the clinician's office extending it to situations where it matters.

These four conditions, which are central to established exposure protocols developed by Edna Foa and colleagues, have clear implications for the session. We don't begin exposure exercises before we have reviewed the model with a patient, collaborated with him or her to develop and initial exposure exercise, and explained to him or her how completing such a personalized exercise helps attain his or her goal of overcoming his or her fears (use the checklist in Box 3.2 to assess whether the patient is ready). As clinicians, we must balance the direction we provide by structuring the session to allow him or her to take on the leadership role in his or her change. The patient assumes control by helping fine-tune the exposure exercises in the early stages and initiates and develops new in-session and homework exercises in the later stages of treatment. Perhaps of greatest concern to many clinicians is that exposure therapy can be harmful. Preventing another potentially sensitizing experience requires that we carefully plan the sessions such that exposure practice can be prolonged and repeated. We don't try an exposure exercise with 10 minutes left in the session. Instead, we finish that session early and schedule a new session that is long enough to practice preventing escape and seeing the effects of doing that over and over again.

3.3.4.1. Getting Bored with It

Clinicians often underestimate the necessity and power of repetition. It's true that completing one 5-minute speech in a session is an accomplishment for Jorge. It's particularly impressive if Jorge can also articulate that completing a 5-minute speech was not as bad as he thought. Seeing this initial success coupled with the effort it took to get there may motivate the clinician to end exposure practice for the session. We argue that entering a session with the goal to complete multiple trials sets you up for a more effective and gratifying experience with exposure therapy. Consider, for example, the stair climbing exercise discussed earliest. The overestimation of fear or the violation of harm expectancy ("It wasn't as bad as I thought) evident in the first trial is common and helpful as it illustrates that the process of fear extinction applies to this patient like it does for others. Ending exposure practice for the session with three trials during which the patient experiences no fear is powerful—getting *bored* with a previously feared cue is an unequivocal sign of new safety learning.

There is no better way to cement new safety learning than making what are obvious indicators of success to us clinicians explicit to the patient. Explicit here means showing the data and relating this back to the model.

> Wow, so impressive. I know this was difficult to do. Check out the board (see Figure 3.10). I just graphed both expected SUDs and actual SUDs across the eight trials that you completed. What do you make of it?"

Trial	Expected SUDs	Actual/Peak SUDs
1	40	35
2	35	35
3	35	30
4	30	25
5	25	15
6	15	0
7	15	0
8	0	0

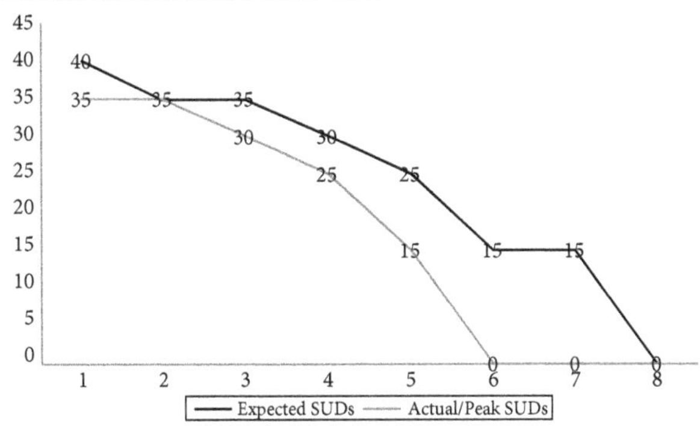

Figure 3.10 Tracking progress during exposure.

3.3.4.2. A Word about SUDs

We use SUDs and their change as one means to judge the success of an exposure exercise—*initial* or *peak* SUDs tell us whether we have established an opportunity for learning, *reductions* in SUDs can point to the fact that new safety learning has occurred (again, provided that the drop in SUDs is not a result of safety behavior utilization), and the discrepancy between *expected/predicted* and *peak* SUDS highlights the process for safety learning by violating harm expectancies. It can be tricky to balance attention to a good exposure practice with modeling adaptive responses to fear (false alarms). That is, when repeatedly asking about SUDs levels during an exposure exercise, you may inadvertently signal to the patient that his or her fear is important and that we need to pay attention to it rather than to let it go.

> It's important for me to be consistent in my messaging during the sessions. I'll be helping you relinquish control when we do these exposure exercises so that you can walk away seeing that you do not have to respond to your fears. They are false alarms and should be treated as such. So, I don't want us to focus too much on SUDs.
>
> I'll ask you for a number in the beginning, just to make sure that we have created the right learning opportunity, and then again later on toward the end of each exercise."

Figure 3.10 depicts a scenario that illustrates that the planning of exposure can result in the expected activation of fear and that simple repetition engenders the decline of SUDs consistent with fear extinction. Sometimes, however, initial or peak SUDs are much lower than expected. When this discrepancy is not better explained by the use of safety behaviors (i.e., the patient actively attempted to fight or manage the fear) or a mismatch (e.g., "I thought I would blush but I didn't"; "Traffic was much lighter, allowing me to keep moving"), such discrepancy can be a welcoming surprise. Indeed, this "prediction error" can be processed as an index of safety learning.

3.3.5. Facilitating Learning during Exposure Practice: In-Exercise Strategies

All of us recognize that the simple act of reading doesn't necessarily result in the acquisition of new knowledge. Learning and retaining new information requires not just attention and concentration but also a way of productively engaging with the material that is presented. This principle holds true for the new safety learning that can occur during exposure therapy as well. There is a reason why we favor in-session or clinician-guided exposure, or at least starting with that, over relying solely on patient-guided exposure. As clinicians, we can observe the approach the patient takes to learning during exposure practice and provide immediate feedback to fine-tune their style and, thereby, optimize outcomes.

Attending to a successful learning experience with exposure practice and preparing to possibly intervene requires that we as clinicians periodically, during exposure practice, ask ourselves at least the following two questions:

(1) Is the patient "relaxing" with the fear?
(2) Is the patient effectively addressing the "what if" questions?

Relaxing with the fear doesn't imply that we want patients to focus their attention and actions on feeling more calm during exposure. As we have discussed, going about exposure in that way, which often matches the patient's preferences, likely has paradoxical effects. Relaxing with the fear simply means that we would like for our patients to act—both in terms of their thinking and their behavioral strategies—in a manner that is consistent with safety. If we observe that Jorge, for example, continues to pace around, wring his hands, and frequently checks the clock on the wall during his repeated speech exposure practice, it's possible that, despite engaging in exposure practice, Jorge is starting to view the cue as more aversive and threatening as opposed to more benign. This is a time to intervene.

> As your coach, I am always thinking about how I can optimize your training experience. You know that our mission is for you to see that performing in front of others is not that meaningful. You will get there with repeated practice. I know, though, that we can speed this up if we carefully line up your actions during practice with the mission, so getting you to act in a way that clearly signals *this is not a big deal*. To figure out what that looks like for you, I think it would be helpful if you could tell me and maybe show me how a Jorge who doesn't care so much would act in this situation."

Identifying the differences between a Jorge who is fighting the anxiety and a Jorge who relaxes with the fear helps generate clear and measurable additional goals (that can be added to the exposure planning worksheet) during subsequent trials (e.g., leaning against a table, smiling, and/or letting his eyes wander around the room while giving the speech).

A patient, after learning unconditional safety or effectively addressing the "what if" questions, is creative and offers ideas about how to change the parameters of the exposure exercise. Seeing this type of initiative develop in a patient over the course of sessions is a sign that exposure therapy is going well—that patient has embraced the model and is taking charge of his or her change. Many patients, though, tend to be careful, not wanting to rock the boat too much, especially early in the intervention. In doing so, they inadvertently weaken the potency of the new safety memory. Their sense of safety remains ambiguous, thus setting these patients up for continued false alarms.

The sigh of relief after an exposure exercise is one potential marker for failing to address critical "what if" questions. Obviously, exposure practice is hard work, and it's understandable if a patient indicates at the end of practice that he or she is glad to be able to shift his or her attention to something that takes less effort. Not to worry if that is indeed the sentiment behind the sigh. The expression of joy or excitement following exposure practice is maybe reserved for few patients, but the fact that this can and does happen makes clear that exposure practice is most powerful and rewarding—and thus more likely to be repeated—when the patient is convinced that what they experienced previously were in fact false alarms. So, it's prudent to assess the meaning of the sigh or any other reactions that appear to signal relief at the end of exposure practice. Consider, for example, that Jorge reports he was happy to see that he was becoming less fearful with each 45-second trial of stair climbing, but at the same time relieved that the practice had ended: He had noticed that there was a large group entering the building, and he was concerned that experiencing all the bodily sensations with others present would feel unsafe and perhaps result in a panic attack. This session would end better if Jorge would be willing to complete some additional trials but this time being the center of attention surrounded by strangers, simply to disconfirm his expectation of a negative and harmful outcome.

Attending to the "what if" questions is acknowledging that learning of safety is context dependent, and recognizing that establishing a robust and clinically meaningful safety memory requires that the clinician and patient make a habit of repeating exposure practice across different contexts. That is, the patient completes practice in the presence of safety cues (e.g., the clinician, when he or she is not stressed or fatigued, during a sunny day, with important people close to her, having access to his cell phone) but will not be satisfied until he or she feels safe confronting the fear cue without safety cues and behaviors (e.g., being alone, while it is dark outside, without access to his cell phone or rescue medications).

3.4. Processing of Exposure Therapy

Rehearsal, rehearsal, rehearsal. As soon as exposure practice ends, we shift our focus as clinicians from the acquisition to the retention of learning. Having generated and optimized an experience that shapes a new memory for the patient—one that associates feared and avoided cues with relative safety as opposed to danger—we now must try to do everything we can to help make sure that this memory sticks. Remind yourself that what seems so clear and evident to you ("Surely he's now convinced that racing heart does not cause a heart attack") is likely not apparent to the patient—in this case, Jorge—particularly early on in the intervention. He needs to see it again several times before he no longer believes it is too good to be true. As you assess whether you're on track making exposure therapy a success for your patient, check whether you are committed to promoting rehearsal practice and ensuring its uptake. You perform this assessment at the end of each session, in-between sessions, and at the beginning of the subsequent session.

3.4.1. End-of-Session Processing

Our job at the at the end of the session is to make salient and explicit the discrepancy between what the patient expected to happen and what actually happened during practice. Keeping in mind that feelings or emotions tend to color perceptions and thus the patient's take away can be negatively biased ("I didn't go very well because I was so anxious"), we are most effective in achieving this aim if we use the Socratic method central to cognitive therapy developed by Aaron Beck. We start with a general open-ended question and then follow up with a series of questions that force the patient to consider the objective evidence allowing him or her to arrive at the conclusion that his or her predictions are exaggerated. The following sequence of questions would likely be useful at the end of Jorge's session, which has been illustrated in Figure 3.10:

- "That was an amazing effort you put in today. I am very excited about that. Now, tell me in your own words—as in if you were going to summarize this for a friend—what you are going to take away from your practice today?" (This question aims to guide the patient to articulate that repeated practices leads to fear extinction and that his threat appraisals are false.)
- "I am reviewing the top of the planning worksheet, which indicates that you were concerned about having a heart attack. Did you experience a heart attack today?" (This question highlights the obvious, which aids threat reappraisal.)
- "The expected fear ratings, particularly in the early trials, were higher than the actual fear ratings. What do you make of this pattern?" (This question aims to help the patient recognize he or she tends to overestimate fear and threat.)
- "It seems to me that your tendency to overestimate threat and fear has some clear implications for how you plan your daily activities. Can you tell me how these overestimations may get in the way?" (This question aims to help

the patient see that his avoidance tendencies are misguided, motivating him to alter his actions.)

- "So, you have learned a few things today about the validity of your predictions and how you can go about correcting these, helping you get rid of the panic and anxiety you experience. Tell me what is useful about these new insights? How will this come in handy as you go into your next week?" (These questions aim to help the patient start thinking about leveraging the in-session learning to make changes to real-life activities [e.g., reducing safety behaviors, starting new activities, developing homework exercises].).

3.4.2. Assigning Homework

We know that relying solely on in-session practice results in a longer course of therapy than when we effectively complement in-session with out-of-session practice. By simply rehearsing activities, homework practice strengthens the learning of the previous session, allowing the patient and clinician to build upon rather than simply repeat activities completed in the previous session. Because homework practice, by definition, takes place in a different context (e.g., outside the clinician's office, without the clinician present, in the presences of other people, in situations that have been linked to false alarms, different time of the day, etc.), it can also further boost the learning of unconditional safety ("Anticipated negative outcomes do not occur no matter how I feel, where I am, what time I am there or who is with me"; see Chapter 2 for a discussion on the importance of varying context when developing new safety memories).

Presenting the rationale for homework practice is easy. We tell our patients that the time spent in the weekly session(s) only represents a very small fraction of our waking hours (approximately only 1%) every week, and thus a patient who makes learning a priority must devote time between sessions to capitalize on the session experience. The reality is, though, that many patients have busy lives and report time constraints. Some even have difficulty fitting in the sessions. Hence, we must anticipate that, despite the right intentions, patients are more likely than not noncompliant to simple homework practice instructions. How do you optimize the prescription?

3.4.2.1. Anticipate

Especially at the beginning of therapy when the patient has not been fully socialized to exposure therapy and has not seen or experienced the positive relation between input and output, the default for patients is limiting the work to the session. We start the assignment of homework with a brief assessment of where the patient is with respect to his or her confidence that he or she can devote meaningful time to rehearsal outside the session.

> You've told me that your work is quite demanding for you, during the day and often also at nights and on weekends. And then you want to spend time with your loved ones. As I am thinking about your busy life, I am wondering how you can fit in practice as it relates to the work that you and I do together. I don't feel good about just winging the homework practice prescription—like deciding on an exercise for practice and then letting you figure out on your own this week when you are going to do this. I've done that before, and often that is unsuccessful. Thus, I would rather develop a specific plan that you feel confident you can complete given the other demands on your time. Can we pull up your calendar, so we can schedule some time slots for practice for the upcoming week?

The guiding principles for effective homework practice are no different from that discussed for in-session exposure exercise. The patient receives the most benefit if the practice completed between sessions is systematic, deliberate, repeated, and prolonged. Thus, the goal is setting aside chunks of time reserved for purposeful practice of a specific exercise, which allows for repetition within the practice session and across practice days/sessions. And, more is better.

3.4.2.2. Balance

We cannot underestimate the advantage of clinician-guided over self-guided exposure practice. In addition to being able to tweak the exposure exercise such that it yields optimal outcomes, the clinician is a safe person motivating the patient to find the courage to persist. Keeping this in mind, we must be prepared to have a discussion about balancing the most effective and potent exposure prescription with one that is feasible and likely to be completed. The principles discussed earlier apply here as well. Specifically, we start ambitiously developing the ideal exposure exercise for home practice—one that can provide the much needed replication and extension (to real life). We must deviate, however, when the patient reports low confidence in being able to complete the ideal exercises.

> I know we agree that hitting the stairwell in your office building every day would nicely build on the work that we have done in session today. The goal is for you to get there and ultimately see that as an activity that is just boring. You're not really confident though that you will be able to do that since I will not be present and you may run into some colleagues. Let's see if we can come up with an intermediary step—an exercise that, when completed, reinforces what you learned today and raises your confidence to do some stairclimbing in your office building next week. And, in doing that, let's see how we can make

it an exercise that also comes with some additional rewards. That is, if possible, I prefer an exercise that gives you opportunity to both learn safety and see how returning to avoided activities brings experiences that make life more fulfilling.

3.4.2.3. Check

We all know how effective a buddy system is when we try to adopt a new routine. Many patients tend to do better with therapy and homework when they sense that their clinicians are there to hold them accountable. Therefore, rather than scheduling the first check on homework practice for the beginning of the following session, which may have the unintended consequence that the patient completes only the practice the day before the session, we recommend repeated checks during the week. A brief message (e-mail, text, or phone as per preference) on the day of the scheduled practice provides the little push that many patients appreciate as they try to figure out how make homework practice a habit.

3.4.2.4. Reward

The ultimate payoff of homework practice is symptom reduction and a return to a more fulfilling life. The distance in time between the effort it takes to complete the homework and this type of reward may be too great for it to motivate the patient to choose homework practice over all the other available activities that provide immediate reward. Competing effectively with easy and enjoyable activities (e.g., watching TV, reading a book, spending time with friends, etc.) thus requires that we enhance the rewarding properties of the homework practice. We can use several easy-to-implement strategies to this end:

- We make an effort to explicitly praise the patient (during checks and sessions) and can encourage that supporting friends or family members do so following the exercise.
- We develop positive contingencies—a list of rewards (e.g., activities, gifts, etc.) that the patient can "give to himself or herself" following successful completion of an exercise.
- We schedule homework practice prior to scheduled activities that are rewarding.

3.5. Treatment Progression

Following the coaching analogy, laying out the focus and content of subsequent "training" sessions all depends on the patient's progress in terms of acquiring and retaining the new safety memory: Is the memory strong, and how can we make sure that we retain that strength and further build on it? Early on in therapy, we may concentrate on the factors that facilitate learning, like enhancing the patient's confidence in therapy and his or her ability to persist in the face of fear along with a sense of safety around previously feared situations, whereas later on in therapy much of our focus is on continuing to push the envelope to providing evidence for unmistakable safety. The ultimate success of therapy becomes evident when the patient has (re)turned to engagement in activities that are consistent with his or her values and chooses activities not based on fear but rather on preferences.

As we detail further in Chapter 4, ongoing assessment provides guidance on the appropriate targets for the session. Specifically, we expect improvements on measures that tap threat appraisals; the trajectory of change in both total scores and individual item scores gives us a sense of whether in-session and homework practice make a dent. Similarly, we ask patients to fade safety behaviors and return to or initiate actions that are consistent with their values. When weekly assessment indicates that progress in these areas is slow or has stalled, we assess the factors that explain progress (e.g., threat appraisals, motivation). These assessment strategies and their outcomes help us identify clear targets for subsequent sessions. This personalized approach to treatment progression makes clear that, although the typical exposure therapy intervention involves 15 to 20 sessions (see Chapters 5–7 for examples of the prototypical intervention), the number of sessions, the sequencing of exercises, and the rate of progression vary across patients and will be guided by the case formulation–driven goals and the success you experience attaining these.

Consider a possible treatment protocol for the case of Jorge (see Table 3.3). It may take two or three sessions to set the stage for exposure practice; these

Table 3.3 Projected Treatment Progression for Jorge

Session	Aims	Activities
1	• Establish diagnosis • Develop initial case formulation	• Assessment
2	• Refine case formulation • Socialize patient to exposure therapy	• Assessment • Education
3–5	• Socialize patient to exposure practice • Experience initial success with exposure practice	• Develop initial exercise • Practice initial exercise
6–11	• Building the safety memory	• Exposure practice
12	• Termination	• Review progress

Box 3.5 Exposure Planning Worksheet Targeting Distress Intolerance

Patient: *Jorge* **Date:** *1-13-2017*

Target threat appraisals (use response on *the ASC and PAI-2*):
Feared outcome: *being perceived as incompetent* Rating: 80%
Feared outcome: Rating:
Feared outcome: Rating:
Feared outcome: Rating:

Goals
Completing a task while experiencing moderate fear (SUDs level of 45), prevent escape.

Situation/Cue
☐ Social interaction:
☐ Social performance: *giving a speech*
☐ Bodily sensation(s): *racing heart*
☐ Other cue(s):

Manipulations to Achieve Match to Fear Cues
☐ Interaction/performance topic: your job
☐ Duration (specify minutes): undetermined
☐ Fade other safety cues/behavior (s) (use response on *the SAFE and TSMQ*):
List targeted safety cue/behaviors:
☐ Induction of interoceptive sensations (list):
☐ Social errors/mishaps (specify):
☐ Feedback:

Set specific and achievable behavioral goal (based on goals and manipulations):
Complete a presentation about your job of undetermined length (speech will be stopped by me rather than a drive to escape).
In front of me and a camera (allowing notes and 5-minute preparation and no audience).

Notes: ASC = Appraisal of Social Concerns scale; PAI-2 = Panic Appraisal Inventory-2; SAFE = Subtle Avoidance Frequency Examination; TSMQ = Texas Safety Maneuvers Questionnaire.

sessions focus on assessment and education to (a) establish diagnoses; (b) develop a personalized fear profile with specific targets for practice; and (c) ensure that Jorge knows what to expect from exposure therapy both in terms of the procedures and its effects. The two to three sessions that follow can aim to get further buy-in from Jorge. The initial exposure practice centered on feared bodily sensations (see Box 3.4 and Box 3.5) provides evidence that (a) repeatedly leaning into false alarms helps turn off the alarm system ("I notice that I can get bored with this cue") and (b) predictions of harm are false ("I have done this several times and nothing bad has happened"). Subsequent practice can then focus on strengthening the safety memory by attending to and addressing the "what if" questions that limit the generalization of in-session learning to progress in real life. The objective of early sessions may be to vary "internal" contexts (e.g., fear and related sensations, stress) during practice, while later sessions can seek to re-establish a sense of safety across "external" contexts (e.g., people, places, time of day) without using safety behaviors (e.g., checking pulse or exits, preparation for social interaction and performance situations; see Figure 3.4). Treatment with Jorge may be terminated when he no longer experiences false alarms, has learned to relate differently to anxiety ("False alarms do not dictate my actions"), and is starting to (re)turn to valued-driven activities.

3.6. Conclusions

In this chapter, we have described the general approach to delivering exposure therapy. We have made clear that assessment and case formulation guide goal-setting and drive the development of exposure exercises, the decisions of what to do in the session, and how to progress. In the chapters that follow, we detail how to assess success (Chapter 4) and provide specific considerations for implementing this approach for common fear cues including emotions and related physical sensations (Chapter 5), people (Chapter 6), and thoughts, images, and traumatic memories (Chapter 7), as well as when patients present for exposure therapy and also take medications (Chapter 8).

4
Assessing Success

4.1. Overview

So far in this book, we have described the principles and procedures of a personalized approach to exposure therapy. Rather than a blanket prescription that ignores individual differences in the presentation and maintenance of anxiety, we have argued that clinicians and patients will be more effective with exposure therapy when they use the case formulation to guide the development and implementation of interventions. Inherent to this individualized therapy approach is the belief that success in exposure therapy requires effectively targeting the key maintaining factors—that is, the learned associations to fear cues that explain why false alarms recur and have persisted over time. We are successful when we have helped the patient develop new associations (memories) of safety in relation to these fear cues.

This chapter is concerned with the ongoing assessment of progress: Deciding in the context of each session whether treatment is on track. The "yardsticks" by which this session-by-session progress is measured is deserving of particular attention, in part because it represents a translation of the patient's goals into safety-learning markers of this process. Certainly, patients have their long-range goals clear for treatment: They want to get rid of symptoms and see an improvement in functioning and quality of life (see Figure 4.1).

We as clinicians not only keep the patient's framing of therapy goals in mind, but also translate these goals into the appropriate week-by-week signifiers of progress. Accordingly, we teach our patients that exposure therapy is on track when the patient is:

(1) Approaching his or her feared cues.
(2) Responding differently to the fear, related emotions, and thoughts.
(3) Shifting his or her specific appraisals of threat to appraisals of safety.

So, in addition to measuring the core symptoms and quality of life, we attend to the treatment process (see Figure 4.2) to assess whether we are on track. We monitor the patient's actions during the sessions (see Figure 4.3); for example, is he or she engaging in exposure practice, is he or she relinquishing control, and is he or she processing disconfirmatory evidence. Likewise, between sessions, we are

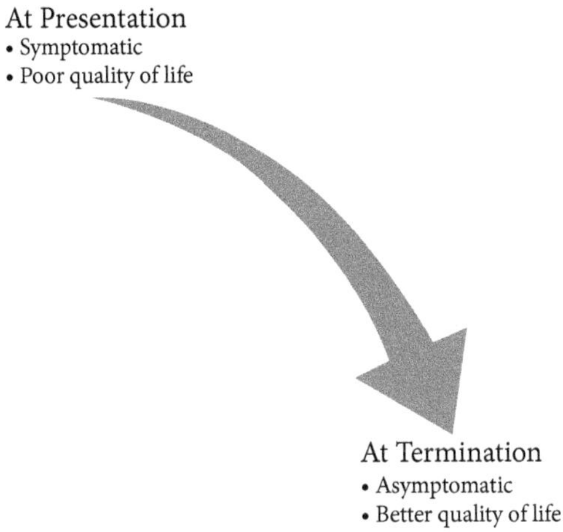

Figure 4.1 Success from the patient's perspective.

attentive to the regularity of sessions, patient preparation for the sessions, completion of therapy homework, and the patient's active discussion and evaluation of this homework. This type of assessment provides us with an idea as to whether the patient is receiving an adequate "dose" of exposure therapy. In other words, when a patient is not seeing symptom improvement (and we see no reason to modify the case formulation), it's a fair assumption that we are underdosing the patient. Underdosing here refers to suboptimal engagement in the core processes of exposure therapy; that is, the patient received the pill but the pill is missing some of the core therapeutic ingredients.

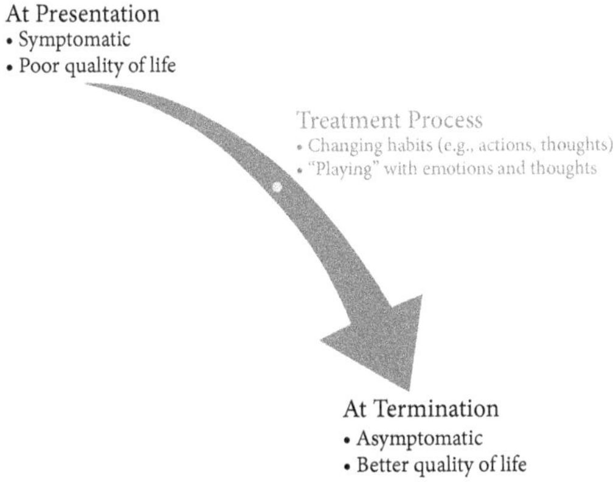

Figure 4.2 Successfully engaging in the process of exposure therapy.

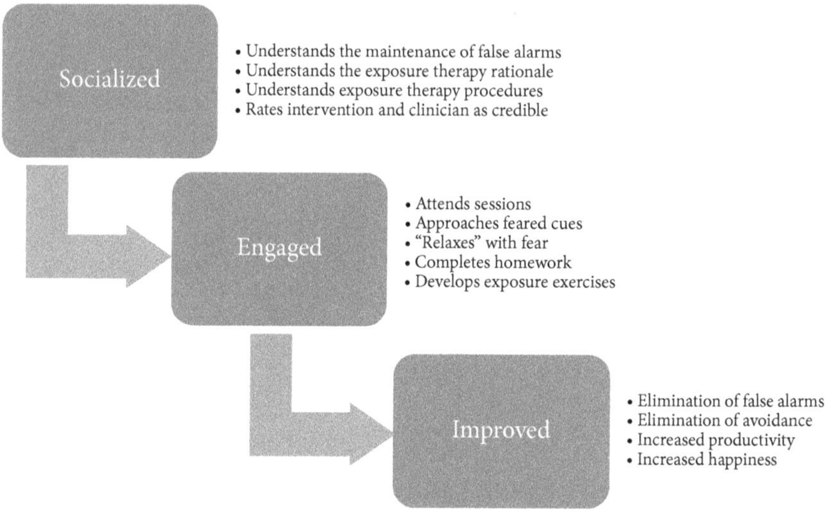

Figure 4.3 Yardsticks for success by domain.

When we are underdosing, we may end up increasing the actual therapy dose (e.g., number of sessions, length of sessions, frequency of sessions), but often suboptimal engagement is a result of poor socialization to treatment. Accordingly, this suboptimal engagement will not be resolved with more sessions unless we attend to socialization (see Figure 4.3). Early in treatment, we may simply ask the patient to articulate what maintains his or her false alarms and how exposure therapy can be used to target the maintaining factors. Later in the intervention, we turn more to the patient for his or her input when setting session targets and deciding on how to best intervene. When a patient successfully participates in these activities (i.e., he or she thinks like a clinician), we know he or she is socialized to exposure therapy.

4.2. Approach

At all stages of the intervention, attending to success requires that we stay process-oriented rather than strategy-oriented. We don't approach sessions like a technician who simply focuses on completing a set of predetermined activities. Instead, we approach the session with a learning objective and conclude that that the session is successful if the patient has attained the learning we set out for the session, *regardless* of the activity. The general learning objective of exposure therapy is establishing a new safety memory. In this section, we will review the learning objectives and corresponding indices of success by stage of the intervention, beginning at the initial contact and ending at treatment termination. This provides a method for attending to and revising the case formulation at each stage of therapy.

4.2.1. Early Sessions

During initial meetings (e.g., phone call, intake evaluation, early sessions; see Chapter 3), the central aim is to develop an initial case formulation and corresponding personalized treatment plan. We are doing that right when the patient can articulate the core themes/thoughts (i.e., threat appraisals) that drive the his or her fear and has identified the actions (i.e., safety behaviors, escape, and avoidance) that maintain the perceived threat–fear relation. A self-assessment check for the clinician on the adequacy of case formulation is that we find the false alarms the patient is experiencing sensible given his or her thinking and actions: "Anyone who would have these thoughts and/or behaved in that way would experience these false alarms."

While the clinician attends to the case formulation and treatment planning, the patient is on his or her own journey with regard to the conceptualization of therapy. This journey undoubtedly concerns a cost–benefit analysis of therapy and the clinician. Costs include the time and financial investments in therapy as well as the emotional investments (talking about and doing anxiety-provoking things). Part of the patient's socialization of therapy is developing a frame that says these investments are likely to be worthwhile. This evaluation process includes estimates of both the coherence of the intervention model as well as the competence of the clinician. A patient frame of "This clinician knows what he is doing," as well as "This clinician will deliver an intervention that is effective," should enhance the patient's willingness to engage fully in exposure exercises. Yet, as important as these attributions are for enhancing openness to the new experiences brought by exposure therapy, early understanding of the model of exposure (e.g., "I am going to use exposure to try out new ways to react to the things that scare me and to find out how it goes under these new conditions") is even more important. Early understanding of the model of exposure therapy indicates that the patient is becoming an important co-clinician on the case, helping guide effective interventions both in and out of sessions. In short, we believe a patient is more likely to continue his or her personal investments in therapy when feeling a strong connection to therapy and is socialized to the exposure therapy model. This is when we see evidence that the patient has begun to take the initial steps in becoming his or her own clinician.

Getting a patient to co-pilot the intervention requires that he or she fully understands how we view false alarms and how we use exposure therapy to effectively treat them. Box 4.1 provides guidance on how to assess success in this domain and implies that we as clinicians have to stimulate collaboration and encourage participation.

> As I have been saying, this is a learning-based treatment. Every session is about acquiring new knowledge, which then will be cemented into long-term memory as you complete the follow-up exercises at home. I think that concept (i.e., coming to a session to learn something new and then practice that learning in-between sessions) is maybe different from how most people think about psychotherapy. You'll see that we will be setting an agenda each session, and although the agenda will list activities, we will emphasize the goals of the activities. For example, today, the session would be considered successful if you left having a better understanding of why it is that you continue to have these panic attacks.
>
> This concept of thinking about the session as a time to learn also implies that you will be active, helping me fine-tune the exposure exercises such that you can get the most out of them. For you to be able to start co-piloting the sessions,

Box 4.1 Assessing Success in Socialization

The patient recognizes

- ❑ That threat appraisals fuel the cue–anxiety/panic relation.
- ❑ That an appraisal of immediate threat produces panic whereas an appraisal of future threat produces anxiety.
- ❑ That anxiety and panic serve a protective function.
- ❑ That avoidance or escape are natural responses to anxiety/panic.
- ❑ The difference between a true an false alarm.
- ❑ That safety behaviors in response to a false alarm maintain the cue–threat appraisal–anxiety/panic relation.

The patient understands

- ❑ That exposure exercises are designed to re-establish a sense of safety around the feared cues.
- ❑ That exposure therapy differs from exposure in real life (deliberate, systematic, prolonged, repeated).
- ❑ That preventing safety behavior use during exposure is critical to developing the new memory of safety.
- ❑ That exposure exercises are successful when he or she does not "fight" the anxiety but instead learns to "relax" with/do nothing about it.
- ❑ That the design of exposure exercises will be done collaboratively.

you need start thinking about anxiety and fear differently, how you may be able to play with these emotions to become more comfortable reacting differently to the things that currently induce fear. Obviously, it will take some time to get you up to speed, but as we move through the sessions, I will be looking to more and more for your input and initiative."

4.2.2. During Exposure Practice

Our ideal is for clinicians to enter the sessions with a plan for how to structure exposure practice to enhance safety learning and then work with the patient to implement it well against the changing backdrop of the patient's mood, motivations, and idiosyncratic reactions to the cues to be presented. Once the patient has started the exposure exercise, how can we tell if it's going well? Rating success of exposure practice requires monitoring of several dimensions

4.2.2.1. Patient's Actions

Does the patient engage in the actions that facilitate safety learning?

(1) The patient attends to the feelings and sensations, as in he or she can label these experiences and is willing to accept their presence (as opposed to fighting/avoiding them).
(2) The patient relinquishes attempts to control symptoms by engaging in safety behaviors and other efforts to short-circuit the fear.
(3) The patient engages in actions that signal safety, as in he or she modifies his or her posture, for example (ensuring it is consistent with safety), and is willing to take "risks," as in he or she pushes the envelope demonstrating that harm is unlikely (e.g., he sprints when he's afraid of having a heart attack; she makes a mistake on purpose when she is concerned about negative evaluation, etc.)

4.2.2.2. Clinician's actions

Does the clinician help ensure the saliency of safety (information)?

(1) The clinician is excited about planning the exercise and is calm during the exercise, communicating that, although recognizing the patient experiences fear and expressing empathy, he or she is not concerned about harm.
(2) The clinician attends to objective markers of true safety, as exemplified by repeatedly asking the patient whether harm has occurred.
(3) The clinician highlights the discrepancy between anticipated and actual outcomes.

4.2.2.3. Another Word about SUDs

It's clear that a decline in the patient's fear ratings (e.g., Subjective Units of Distress Scale [SUDs]) marks the reacquisition of a sense of safety. Once a patient can approach a previously feared cue with a SUDs level near zero without engaging in any safety behaviors, he or she is no longer expecting harm; that is, he or she has succeeded in getting bored with the exercise and the related cues. Hence, a reduction of SUDs is an index of success. We are aware, though, of concerns that have been raised about relying on SUDs ratings as a yardstick of improvement in exposure therapy. We will list two frequently mentioned concerns and our ideas of how to address them next.

(1) *Patients are not good at using the SUDs rating scale to rate the intensity of fear.* Some have argued that the SUDs ratings we obtain from patients appear either random (i.e., patients just pick a number to appease the clinician and the process) or not reflective of their fear levels (i.e., patients rate SUDs higher or lower than they actually feel). This observation, which definitely holds for some patients in our experience, simply implies that patients need to be trained on how to use SUDs and we need to keep an eye on calibration as needed. During the initial sessions, we introduce the SUDs rating scale (see Figure 4.4) and complete a brief exercise to ensure that ratings accurately reflect their feelings.

> To give us a sense of how we are doing with the exposure practice, we need to get an idea of how much fear you experience and whether that fear changes during and with practice. The scale we use is called the Subjective Units of Discomfort Scale or SUDs scale. Let's take a look at the scale and get you comfortable with the ratings. As you can see, there are descriptive labels at zero, 25, 50, 75, and 100. Obviously, you will be selecting any number between zero and 100—like 73, 51, 11, or 5—so don't limit it to these five numbers. But, I do want to review the labels with you to make sure that your ratings accurately capture how you feel. So, let's start by giving me a SUDs rating reflecting the level of fear that you experience now?

SUDS–Distress, Anxiety, or Emotional Discomfort

0 5 10 15	20 25 30 35 40	45 50 55 60 65	70 75 80 85 90	95 100
No anxiety, calm, relaxed	Mild anxiety, alert, able to cope	Moderate anxiety, some trouble concentrating	Severe anxiety, thoughts of leaving	Very severe anxiety, extreme fear

Figure 4.4 Subjective Units of Distress Scale.

Once you have an initial SUDs rating, you can begin the initial calibration. You will ask the patient to justify his or her rating using the descriptor provided for the closest anchor, verify its accuracy, and then go on to review the range: That is, SUDs levels that are lower than the current rating and SUDs levels that are higher than the current rating.

> I believe that a SUDs of 20 does capture your current experience well, given that you feel somewhat hyped up and more uneasy than you think is reasonable. Obviously, a zero SUDs score means no fear whatsoever. Can you think of an experience when you felt calm and relaxed or may be even excited and thus had a zero SUDs score?
>
> Let's think about experiences too when you had higher SUDs than now. As you can see, a 50 SUDs is when fear is bothersome and uncomfortable, as in you have some problems concentrating, but at the same time, and this is important, you can cope and are not thinking about escape. Can you describe an experience when your SUDs were 50?
>
> What about a situation when you experienced a SUDs of 75? This would be a time when you felt extremely uncomfortable, had lots of fear sensations, and were having difficulty coping. As in all you could think about is how bad the fear felt and started having thoughts of needing to get out.
>
> Finally, I'd like you to think about the SUDs rating of 100, when fear is overwhelming, your alarm system is fully activated, as in you have intense fear sensations, and you cannot think of anything else but leaving the situation. Can you describe such an experience?"

Part of the socialization process, this brief exercise helps the patient see the importance of a valid SUDs rating and understand the range. This exercise can be repeated in later sessions when the clinician and/or patient believe ratings are off or not in line with the patient's experience.

(2) *Exposure practice can be productive even if SUDs remain high throughout.* Many clinicians who practice effective exposure therapy have had great sessions in which patients ended with high SUDs levels. At first sight, such a statement appears at odds with the idea that a decline in SUDs or a low SUDs level at the end of the session is an index of success. It's true that ending a session with high SUDs ratings provides no evidence for having established a safety memory. If that was the case, SUDs would be zero. In the context of an exposure therapy program (i.e., a number of sessions each consisting of exposure practice), exposure practice that ends with high SUDs can be an index of success, but it depends on the session goals and the postexposure processing. Indeed, when targeting the fear of panic, let's say, the goals of exposure practice

can be inducing panic to learn that panic attacks are harmless (see Chapter 5). In that case, exposure practice will only be successful if SUDs are high. But, in this case and other practices that end with high SUDs, there always is the risk of sensitization (i.e., the patient leaves the session feeling less safe as opposed to more safe when experiencing a panic attack and the related bodily sensation). Thus, when exposure practice ends with high SUDs ratings, postexposure processing focusing on preventing desensitization is important.

> Wow, that was amazing effort on your part. The exercise went exactly as we planned. You experienced an intense false alarm and were able to lean in, sending the message to yourself that, although intense and uncomfortable, there is no threat. I do want to talk some about later today and tomorrow. My experience is that, especially when it's the first time in exposure therapy, a false alarm can be sensitizing to patients. What I mean is that patients sometimes have a hard time not looking back in the hours and days following such an exposure and interpret it as aversive or even a failure. False alarms have affected your life; you come here to get rid of them, so you can't help experiencing some doubt when leaving a session like today's. So, I am not so much concerned about that initial reaction of doubt. I do want to make sure that you respond to that productively, so let's spend a little time developing a strategy."

A productive and effective response to doubt is *recognition, validation*, and *refutation*, and in that order. The goal is to help a patient leave anticipating that his or her fear habit (i.e., thoughts, actions, feelings) will be prominent in the hours and days following an exposure practice ending in high SUDs and that this reaction is normal. This helps prepare the patient to take appropriate action for using the in-session experience to aid in safety learning. That is, rather than being demoralized (e.g., "These sessions are too hard"; "Why am I still thinking about it?"), recognition ("I knew this was coming") and validation ("It makes sense given my fear habit") put the patient in a position to choose a strategy that further weakens the *cue–threat appraisal–action–fear* relation (i.e., refutation) both in terms of his *cognitive* and *behavioral* actions:

Cognitive:

- "This is the bully taunting me; it's best to not fight the negative self-evaluation bully."
- "I know I feel like I failed, but there is no evidence of failure or harm."
- "Do I really want to let my feelings misguide my actions?"
- "This was challenging but not threatening."

Behavioral:

- Engaging in productive action: "What would I do now if I wasn't anxious?"
- Shifting the environment (e.g., moving into a different room, going outside, being around other people) to be able to respond to different cues.

In addition to developing the cognitive and behavioral responses, consider the tools that can help ensure that the patient engages in these responses:

- Enlist the help of the patient's support network that can remind the patient of the appropriate actions and reinforce them.
- Use reminder cues in his or her environment (e.g., sticky notes on the fridge and in the car, phone apps that have reminder features).

As we mentioned before, there are times when, after careful planning of exposure to match a patient's fears, the patient completes the exposure with very low SUDs ratings—no fear to exposure to their fearful stimuli. What to make of this? This is either very good news or a poorly targeted exposure. In the former case, patients' behaviors may have been driven so long by anticipatory anxiety and avoidance that they are surprised to learn that actually facing the avoided situation/cues is far easier than anticipated. In this case, the clinician has achieved the desired discrepancy in expectations as assessed by high anticipatory anxiety followed by relative comfort during exposure and persistence with the fear cues. We believe this profile is more common with those with long-standing avoidance but few recent experiences with their fear cues. Accurate targeting of the exposure is measured by the anticipatory anxiety rather than the SUDs during exposure, and the low SUDS can be taken as quick, reality-based learning that violates the expectancies held by the patient. Good therapeutic learning!

Yet, it is also possible that the exposure was "a miss"—that crucial cues or contexts were missing from the exposure. Determining the true meaning of the exposure (good learning or a miss) is aided by postevent processing focused on helping the patient examine the reason for the violation of his or her anxious expectancies. For example, the therapist may respond as follows:

- Very interesting! We designed an exposure that had a lot of the elements that concerned you, yet you had very low SUDs during the exposure. What do you make of that?
- Great job! You were really comfortable in that exposure, in a surprising way. Are there any things that could have happened during the exposure that would have left you far less comfortable?

- Given what happened today and your comfort with this exposure, how might you want to coach yourself differently next time you are facing these fear cues? (Follow-up question: Do you feel like that is honest coaching, meaning, do you fully believe that coaching, or do you feel like there is a counterargument?]

In asking these questions, the clinician is curious about special cues/contexts that:

(1) Occur internally ("It would have been much harder had my heart started pounding," "I am not sure how I would have done had I thought too much about the fact that people who know me may see me," or "I think I always do better when I am well rested").
(2) Are linked to performance ("I got off to a good start, so I knew I would be fine" or "I just wanted to make a good show because we are out in public").
(3) Are linked to external context ("I knew I would be fine because I am in a hospital clinic; what could happen here?" or "I knew you would intervene if my panic got too bad").

These absent cues/contexts inform the clinician on how to modify subsequent exposure exercises (during the current or a subsequent session) to help patients to expand their sense of safety. Indeed, one important relapse prevention consideration is to ensure that patients are comfortable with their fear cues when anxiety symptoms are present as well as when they are absent. For this reason, part of resilience training for patients is for clinicians to fully enjoy and commend low-SUDs exposure practice while also ensuring that their patients can also complete these exposure exercises when symptoms are present. Hence, clinicians will want to target some exposure exercise while symptoms are induced with the interoceptive exposure strategies. Chapter 5 is devoted to the importance of exposures in the context of anxiety symptoms.

4.2.3. Immediately after Exposure Practice

Especially early on in exposure therapy, patients can't help but feel a sense of relief when practice ends. It's hard to go against a habit especially when there is still doubt as to whether the alarm is false and whether the treatment can be effective. Certainly, you want to validate and normalize these perhaps mixed reactions to exposure practice, but you do want to be sure that it doesn't take away from cementing therapeutic learning.

Successful end-of-session processing is evident when the patient communicates that the session clarified

(1) That he or she suffers from false alarms.
(2) The discrepancy between anticipated harm and actual harm.
(3) The utility of repeated exposure to fear cues.
(4) The utility of fading out safety behaviors and leaning into the feelings produced by false alarms.

In addition to facilitating a take-home message that is therapeutic, you want to ensure that the patient relates the new learning to subsequent out-of-session experiences. That is, we aim not only to begin re-establishing a sense of safety around fear cues in the session but also recognize that real gains are made with respect to forming new safety memories when the patient applies the approach taken in the session to situations as they occur in real life.

> Let's talk about how you can capitalize on the learning that took place during the session today. It's incredible to me that you are able to put in so much effort. Your alarm system goes off, which directs you to escape, yet you stayed in there, leaned in, and let the fear run its course. Obviously, it was worth it, as you learned your concerns about harm are invalid. What's important now is that you can take what you did in the session and apply this to situations as they present themselves over the next week. Can we talk a little bit about your upcoming week, the situations you anticipate will be challenging, and how you might go about these reinforcing what you learned today?"

4.2.4. At the Beginning of the Session

From the perspective of the clinician practicing exposure therapy, the days prior to the session have gone well if the patient has

(1) Noticed an improvement in fear and related symptoms.
(2) Noticed he or she has started "relating" differently to his or her feelings, thoughts, and actions.
(3) Approached fear cues as per the homework assignment.

These indices of success include outcomes (i.e., the main goal of treatment), processes (i.e., the path to achieving the main goal), and strategies (i.e., the methods required to engage the therapeutic process). They are not independent. We know that achieving an improvement in symptoms requires that patients relate differently to the feelings, thoughts, and actions that occur when they approach fear cues. Importantly, though, there can be a delay between engaging in therapeutic actions (e.g., approaching fear cues, leaning into fear) and experiencing a consistent improvement in symptoms. In fact, it is not uncommon that a patient reports a slight worsening in symptoms in the beginning of exposure therapy or when he or she and the clinician push the envelope on exposure practice. This worsening simply is a result of removing safety behaviors and will be temporary when the patient and clinician ensure that the patients remains persistent in his or her actions—that is, leaning in to allow fear to run its course.

Checking in on all three indices at the beginning of sessions reminds the patient and clinician of the goals and thus allows for reinforcement when progress is evident or fine-tuning when progress in any of the three domains is lacking.

> I reviewed the scores on the measures you completed last night, and I am very happy to see that you continue to experience improvements in symptoms. At the end of the session last week, I asked you to summarize what you took away from the exposure exercise and in what way this was useful. You said you learned that you tend to be off in your predictions in terms of being overly concerned that something bad is going to happen, particularly when you are interacting with people at work. Can you tell me how your week was different because of our exposure practice last week?

4.2.5. Termination

As we make clear in the previous chapters, prototypical exposure therapy is about 10 to 15 sessions. Certainly, the time to termination varies across patients and depends on various factors (e.g., core fears, comorbid health and mental health problems, motivation, presence or absence of other stressors) and their combinations. In addition, termination can be premature for reasons such as a change in life circumstances, a change in priorities, or moving to a new locale. Ideally, the patient and clinician agree to terminate because they have successfully achieved therapy goals and believe that additional therapy is not indicated. In the case of exposure therapy, the following indices mark success supporting the decision to terminate:

(1) The patient no longer experiences false alarms when confronted with previously feared stimuli as evident from self-report measures (see Chapter 9) and in-session confrontation with cues.

(2) The patient has greater allegiance to his or her values and no longer avoids safe experiences (e.g., activities, situations, sensations, thoughts, images) because of fear.
(3) The patient has a different relationship with fear, treating anxiety/fear as a signal that may or may not be accurate.

4.3. Conclusions

In this chapter, we have described what we consider the core yardsticks of improvement clinicians want to attend to as they prescribe personalized exposure therapy. We have highlighted the importance of measuring the engagement in treatment and its associated factors, the engagement in the therapeutic learning process, and the main outcomes that both patients and clinicians seek. We refer the reader to Chapter 9 for a list of measures that can facilitate the assessment of success across these domains.

5
Fear of Emotions and Related Physical Sensations

5.1. Overview

This chapter details exposure strategies for fears that underlie and intensify a wide range of disorders: Fears of emotions and related physical sensations. Why do these fears have a broad impact on psychopathology? Quite simply, it is because it is especially hard when the focus of fears is inside one's own body. This is the case with fears of emotional and somatic experiences: The fear lurks within.

In contrast, imagine a world where you are comfortable with your own experience of negative emotions. If you are more comfortable with experience of anticipatory anxiety, every work meeting, every conflict with a coworker or a spouse, and every case presentation at staff meetings will be more comfortable because the experience of anxiety itself does not derail the experience. Likewise, if you able to tolerate a rapid heart rate and feelings of nausea, you will be more likely to engage in high-intensity workouts. Furthermore, if you are more able to tolerate feelings of sadness, you may be better able to talk about the loss of a loved one. And, if you are better able to tolerate feelings of sadness, guilt, or anxiety, you will be less likely to stress-eat in response to any of these emotions. In short, getting comfortable with negative and feared emotions and somatic sensations is not just a treatment for anxiety-related disorders, it is also a broad-based strategy for adding well-being and self-control to life.

All psychotherapies have a role in helping patients get more comfortable with their emotional experiences elicited in and out of session. Clinicians communicate acceptance of these emotions and encourage further emotional expression. For example, clinicians routinely work to normalize patients' emotional experience: "Of course you are feeling sad when . . ." or "It is natural to feel anxious when . . ." Clinicians also routinely link symptoms to life provocations: "I think it was more upsetting than you had imagined when . . ." or "Is it possible that the tightness in your stomach is the result of your concerns that . . ." Interoceptive exposure procedures (systematic exposure to feared or avoided internal stimuli) represent a much more focused and hearty expansion of these efforts, where the learning of comfort in relation to emotional experiences is enhanced by specific and focused practice in the presence of these interoceptive cues.

Fears of emotional experiences and bodily sensations are elements of a broader category of *distress intolerance*. Distress intolerance is a person's perceived or actual capacity to withstand negative emotional or somatic states. People differ not only in a general capacity to withstand emotional or somatic stress but also in their profile of distress intolerance. For example, you may be able to tolerate a sore knee while running but be completely undone by the experience of an irregular heartbeat. In terms of the intensity of sensations, the sore knee may be a stronger sensation, but the irregular heartbeat may set off much more anxiety and self-monitoring, depending on your experiences with and beliefs about these sensations. The same is true of the spectrum of anxiety symptoms (e.g., rapid heart rate, heart palpitations, flushing, queasy stomach, sweating, breathlessness, muscle tightness, sinking sensations, dizziness, trembling, depersonalization) that patients may experience.

Concerning attentional processes, fears drive attention to the most fearful aspect of an experience. For example, if you fear dogs, you are more likely to attend to the teeth and claws of a dog rather than the wagging tail. When this natural tendency is applied to fears of physical sensations, a person may become especially adept at noticing the first signs of a feared emotional or somatic experience. For example, even a subtle sensation of flushing may set off fears of additional symptoms to come. Accordingly, the vigilance to symptoms and other somatic sensations may drive a cycle of anxiety and avoidance and may further define feared emotions and sensations as intolerable.

The ability to tolerate negative emotional and somatic states is a core feature of resilience, where resilience can be understood at the ability to persist adaptively in challenging circumstances. When a person has fears/intolerance of his or her own emotional experience, then every stressful event becomes amplified by concerns about resulting emotions. For example, one of the best predictors of emotional intolerance and the many maladaptive conditions linked to it (e.g., use of alcohol, cigarettes, or other drugs to cope with negative affect; eating in response to negative emotions; avoidance of exercise; degree of functional disability in those with conditions causing pain or dyspnea; the ability to follow through on personal behavioral goals ranging from plans to increase exercising or reduce internet use) is *anxiety sensitivity* (defined as the fear of anxiety-related symptoms due to presumed catastrophic consequences of these symptoms). In addition to predicting these negative health and goal achievement patterns, anxiety sensitivity is elevated across the anxiety and mood disorders and is particularly elevated in panic disorder and posttraumatic stress disorder (PTSD). Anxiety sensitivity also decreases with effective treatment and has been supported as a mechanism of therapeutic improvement in panic-related disorders.

In other words, the tendency to fear your own emotional experience and somatic sensations makes life harder: Fears of one's own emotional experience amplifies the aversiveness of stress and negative emotions, it amplifies the aversiveness of substance withdrawal sensations, it plays a role in illness anxiety disorder and anxiety and mood disorders, and it plays a core role in the etiology and maintenance of panic disorder and PTSD. This chapter is devoted to the use of exposure to treat these fears.

5.2. Interoceptive Exposure

Interoceptive exposure is a core procedure for teaching comfort with negative emotional experiences and related somatic sensations. Interoceptive exposure uses physical and perceptual procedures to mimic the somatic sensations associated with negative emotions and may be combined with other techniques (e.g., use of music, videos, or guided imagery) to enhance the production of specific emotional experiences. The goal is to reintroduce the patient's constellation of feared and avoided emotions/sensations, to allow relearning of a sense of safety in response to these emotions/sensations. In this context, safety means that the experience may not be liked, but that the experience of these emotions and related somatic sensations does not lead to emotional escalation (fear of fear) or avoidance due to anticipated physical, mental, or social harm. In short, interoceptive exposure provides patients with opportunities to eliminate fearful expectations about the meaning and ultimate consequences of their emotional experiences and related symptoms.

5.2.1. Phobic Conditions: Fearing the Cue or Fearing the Cued Fear?

A direct focus on interoceptive fears also provides clinicians with a way to parse phobic experiences into separate elements that can be targeted independently. Consider snake phobias. When a person with a snake phobia is presented with a snake, the immediate aversive consequence is not being bitten by the snake. Instead, the immediate aversive consequence is being "bitten" by the experience of anxiety itself, and avoidance is motivated by this experience. Because of the symptom-driven avoidance, the phobic person does not have a chance to see if there are other ultimate dangers to being around a snake.

Certainly, a person can improve from direct therapeutic exposure to snakes, and this exposure brings with it exposure to anxiety sensations. That is, as the patient progresses through in vivo exposure, he or she is being successively exposed to his or her anxiety experience along the way. Depending on the patient, this anxiety may range from mild anticipatory anxiety to a full panic response. The patient has to tolerate this anxiety long enough to persist in the situation and learn that snakes are not as threatening as expected. In the process of tolerating this anxiety, the patient presumably will learn the valuable lessons that:

(1) anxiety responses can be false alarms, with no link to actual danger, and
(2) it is possible to tolerate this false alarm long enough for it to turn off as the true "safety" of the situation is realized.

In other words, all exposure involves exposure to anxiety sensations themselves. Yet, the specialized interventions of interoceptive exposure allow clinicians to isolate fears of anxiety from fears of other cues, like snakes. For example, a clinician could pretreat a fear of the anxiety response (using interoceptive exposure) before ever exposing the patient to a snake. With the pretreatment of any fears of the anxiety response, the patient then has the opportunity to observe and learn of the true safety of snakes without an overwhelming urge to escape from the induced anxiety itself.

When might a clinician wish to parse up the elements of a phobic experience in this way? We believe that it is valuable whenever fears or avoidance of anxiety symptoms is strong enough that it would slow progress in other cue exposure relevant to the disorder. In short, if a patient is avoiding or having difficulty tolerating exposure because of concerns about the experience of anxiety itself, then it is time for interoceptive exposure.

5.3. The Case of Anna

Fears of somatic sensations may develop from a variety of modeling or other early experiences, and/or they may be intensified due to the experience of strong anxiety, depression, or panic. Consider the case of Anna. Anna has long had fears of illness. Starting in high school, she would repeatedly ask her mother whether she was seriously ill when she had aches are pains in her joints. In her early 20s, after a friend's father was diagnosed with skin cancer, she became especially concerned about her moles, spending hours checking whether they had changed shape or whether she had any odd skin sensations in the area of any moles or skin blemishes. She started going to her dermatologist multiple times per year for skin checks. In her mid-20s she started becoming more concerned about illness symptoms more generally after she had an episode of mild tachycardia. She began to monitor her heart rate more closely and became more convinced something was wrong. During one such monitoring episode, she became so frightened by her rapidly increasing heart rate she started experiencing panic symptoms (e.g., rapid breathing, dull chest pain, numbness and tingling around her mouth and scalp, and difficulty focusing her vision/derealization). She called her primary care physician and received assurances that the event was likely anxiety and was seen for an office visit the next day. Nonetheless, Anna's vigilance to her body increased dramatically, and regular panic attacks soon followed. She says that these attacks come out of the blue much of the time, but she also is aware that she has become avoidant of situations where she is concerned about having an attack (in lines in stores, the hairdresser, any long drives). Her primary care physician has recommended treatment with a benzodiazepine (clonazepam) combined with an antidepressant (sertraline), but she is worried about the effects of medication on her body. She has heard about exposure therapy and is willing to try this "more natural" therapy.

5.3.1. Explaining Anna's Presenting Problems

Anna's case represents a subtype of panic disorder that emerges from hypochondriacal concerns. According to case studies and theoretical accounts, the shift from hypochondriacal concerns to panic disorder is occasioned by the shift from a focus on symptoms that are not arousal-related (knee aches or oddly shaped moles) to those that are arousal related (heart rate). It is the focus on arousal-related sensations that creates a feed-forward cycle between anxious concern, increasing symptoms, and corresponding maladaptive safety behaviors. This feed-forward cycle is at the heart of panic disorder and the fear-of-fear cycle that maintains it.

Figure 5.1 depicts this core cycle. As reflected in the figure, many cases of anxiety arise in individuals with a pre-existing history of anxiety difficulties. For example, in clinical samples, we have found that roughly half of patients had a childhood history of anxiety disorders (e.g., overanxious disorder). But this means that half of patients do not have this history. For example, consider the case of James who had panic emerge in his middle 40s at a time of particular job stress. At that time, his uncle, to whom he felt particularly close, had recently had a heart attack. The sudden reality of heart troubles occurring in the family led him to direct extra attention to his own heart and chest symptoms. In short, his job stress had led to both heart palpitations and sternum pain, but with the new interpretive bias provided by his uncle's heart attack, these symptoms now gave him the fear of impending death. His stress symptoms quickly escalated into recurrent panic attacks and increasing avoidance of any activity (e.g., regular exercise) that would seem to "stress" his heart. James's experiences, relative to Figure 5.1, are reflective of the roughly 90% of patients that report onset of panic disorder at a time of stress. The stress provides a backdrop of anxious-arousal symptoms that are subsequently interpreted as dangerous. This perceived

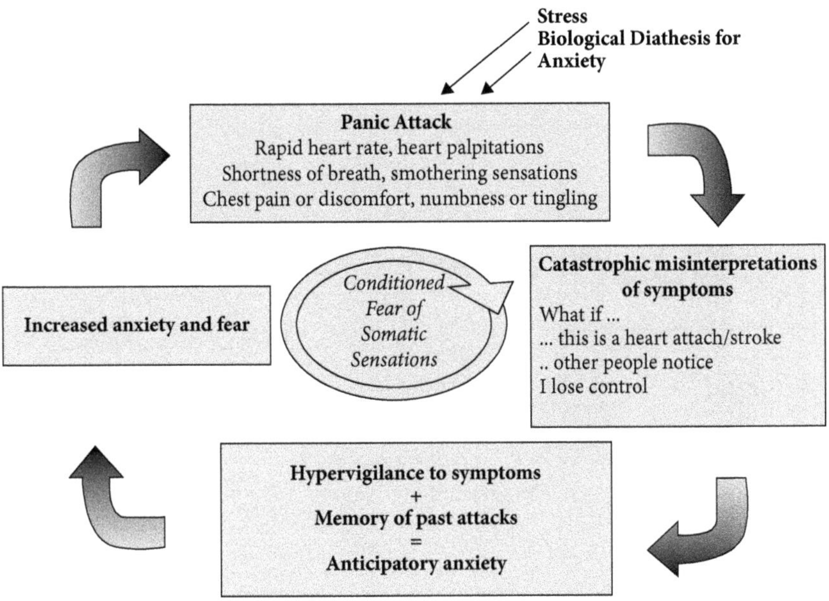

Figure 5.1 The fear-of-fear cycle. Figure adapted from Otto et al., *10-minute CBT*, Oxford, England: Oxford University Press, 2011, p. 52.

dangerousness is heightened by the ongoing cycle of panic, where the recurrent panic attacks set in the sense that something is truly catastrophically wrong with the body.

As noted, the fear of anxiety symptoms also arises from the experience of anxiety and panic itself. The core cycle of Figure 5.1 emphasizes the feed-forward nature of fear-of-fear cycles. Each panic attack is experienced as threatening in own right, typically due to fears that the panic attack denotes (a) threat of death (heart attack, stroke, etc.), (b) threat of loss of control (e.g., "I can't make it through the meeting," "I will crash my car," "I may run amok," etc.), or (c) threat of humiliation or social rejection (e.g., "Others will think I am crazy or defective"). With each recurrence of panic, the sense of being out of control and at risk increases, as does vigilance to and catastrophic interpretations of symptoms. With the strengthening of this cycle, even subtle symptoms of arousal can be interpreted as the start of panic ("Uh oh, I think it is happening now; what if it gets worse?") and can cue additional anxiety and the next panic attack. Accordingly, the cycle of panic ends when the feed-forward cycle is disrupted: To end panic, one first learns not to fear panic sensations.

The feed-forward cycle of panic also arises as part of other disorders and can sap resilience and increase avoidance and disability in those disorders.

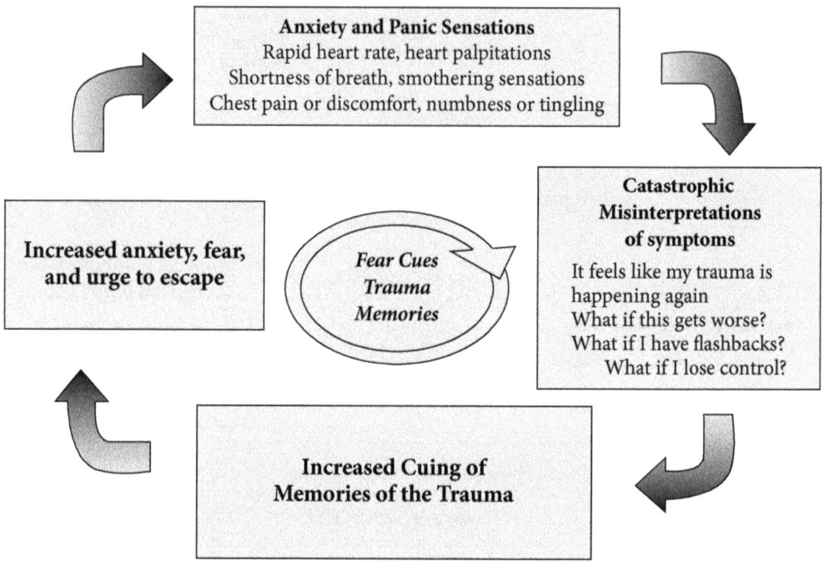

Figure 5.2 The amplification of anxiety and panic sensations in posttraumatic stress disorder.

For example, in PTSD, trauma-related fears include fears of the recurrence of upsetting memories of the trauma as well as the often-overwhelming emotional content linked to the trauma (see Figure 5.2. Indeed, as noted, fears of anxiety symptoms in PTSD are at least as high as those of panic disorder. Because of the prominent role of fears of emotional content of trauma memories ("I can't stand the feelings that come up when I am reminded of my trauma; I feel like I will lose control or be overwhelmed"), fears of symptoms have emerged as an initial target of treatment. That is, much like the previous example of the snake phobic, prior to using exposure to create relative comfort with traumatic memories, interoceptive exposure can be used to promote greater acceptance of the emotions that will be induced by the content-related exposure.

5.4. Assessing the Severity and Profile of Interoceptive Fears

One of the best performing measures of fears of anxiety symptoms and emotional intolerance more generally is the Anxiety Sensitivity Index (ASI; see Chapter 9). We think of this scale as providing a general index of the importance of interoceptive exposure treatment to a patient's functioning. The

ASI-3 is comprised of 18 items encompassing three subdomains: (a) fears of physical sensations (e.g., "It scares me when my heart beats rapidly"), (b) fears of cognitive symptoms (e.g., "When I cannot keep my mind on a task, I worry I might be going crazy"), and (c) fears of social embarrassment (e.g., "It is important to me not to appear nervous"). Each of these items is rated on a 5-point Likert scale and then summed for a total score (0–72). Total cores averaging around the low 30s are common for the panic disorder and PTSD, and scores in the mid-20s are common for depression and the other anxiety-related disorders. Accordingly scores in the mid-20s are indicative, to us, of the need for a specific therapeutic attention to these fears. Yet, the meaning of the overall score is modified by the domain specificity of some of these fears. A patient may have extreme fears in one specific domain or for one specific symptom (e.g., fears of dizziness), but may score low on all other items. Hence, we think a checklist (Table 5.1) is useful for assessment to see if there is specific sensitivity to a particular symptom that leads to disability in daily functioning (see also the Panic Appraisal Inventory in Chapter 9 that can complement this assessment). The ordering of symptoms on this checklist is relevant to the avoidance related disability of the symptoms; that is, not all symptoms have similar effects, and studies have indicated that dizziness and dyspnea engender greater avoidance in people with panic disorder. Hence, these symptoms are placed first in the list. High scores identify the fear of somatic symptoms of anxiety as needing specific attention in the case formulation for your patient.

5.5. Interoceptive Exposure Practice

5.5.1. Generic Approach

Interoceptive exposure procedures have been most developed in relation to symptoms of panic disorder, and Table 5.2 provides a list of common procedures used to elicit panic-like symptoms ranging from derealization and dyspnea to a pounding heart and flushed face. In the most generic application of these procedures, exposure unfolds in five stages:

(1) Patients are told which symptoms are likely to be induced by the procedure (it is true that some protocols for interoceptive exposure attempt to surprise the patient with the symptoms, but we can't see any evidence that these "surprise" elements promote safety learning; we prefer to inform our patients about what is likely to be induced so that the therapeutic attention can be on how the induced symptoms are being interpreted).

Table 5.1 Sensitivity to Somatic and Emotional Experiences Survey

Sensation or Emotion	Applicable YES?	Example of Related Avoidance	Anticipated Threat	Rank Order
Feeling dizzy or faint				
Rapid or irregular heartbeat				
Dyspnea				
Chest pain or pressure				
Dry mouth or difficulty swallowing				
Numbness or tingling				
Face flushing				
Sweating				
Trembling				
Upset stomach or nausea				
Derealization or depersonalization				
Heat or Humidity				
Cold				
Substance withdrawal or craving				
Fatigue				
Sadness				
Boredom				
Guilt				

(2) The symptoms are generated using any of a variety of physical or perceptual procedures to engender symptoms that mimic the emotional and physical experiences of feared sensations. Many of these symptoms are listed in Table 5.2.

(3) Nonphobic responses to these sensations are reviewed/rehearsed in the context of the symptom induction. Concerning this step, if the typical

Table 5.2 Typical Interoceptive Exposure Procedures

Sensations/Emotions Targeted	Procedure
Dizziness, disorientation, and very mild derealization	**Head rolling:** Sitting upright with eyes closed and repeatedly turning the head around in a circle (from midline, around with chin near chest, and then on around to midline)
Dizziness, numbness and tingling (face, scalp, arms), hot flushes	**Hyperventilation:** Breathing one per second with a strong exhale for 60 seconds
Dizziness, disorientation, nausea	**Chair spinning:** Spinning around several times (with eyes closed) in a swivel chair
Rapid heart rate, pounding heart, dyspnea, heavy legs	**Stair running:** Running upstairs or jogging in place
Trembling, numbness/tingling	**Full-body tension:** While seated, tensing forehead and jaw, clenching hands and bring them tightly to the shoulders, pull in the stomach, stress the heals into the floor, clench the toes. Hold for one minute
Chest pressure, sinking feeling in stomach	**Pillow squeeze:** With the arms, tightly squeeze a firm couch pillow to the chest and solar plexus for one minute
Throat tightness, dry mouth	**Rapid swallowing:** Swallowing repeatedly (six swallows) with nothing in the mouth
Visual distortions, derealization	**Hand staring:** Staring intently into the palm for one minute (not allowing the eyes to move to drive distortions in the peripheral visual field (e.g., seeing a finger disappear or an extra finger to appear). **Vision zing:** Staring intently at venetian blinds or any other light/dark stripped array (e.g., office ventilation grate) without moving the eyes for one minute (alternative: staring at any of the many stripped visual illusions available on the Internet)
Flushed face; facial pressure	**Head below knees:** Starting in a sitting lean forward to place the head below the knees for one minute, then rise from that position rapidly (while remaining seated).
Diffuse overarousal: Rapid heart rate, sweaty palms, trembling, anxiety	**Chocolate-covered coffee beans:** Depending on the patient's coffee consumption eating a half dozen beans (or alternatively, rapidly drinking a large coffee) at the start of the session can produce diffuse arousal symptoms that may last for hours

phobic response is to tense up and seek to control the sensations, then the nonphobic response is to *relax with* the symptoms, noticing what they feel like and that they can be experienced safely, if not, ultimately, relatively comfortably. To aid this process, clinicians may need to coach the patient to attend carefully to the sensations induced by the induction and just what is uncomfortable or frightening about these sensations. This is important because some patients will come to treatment after decades of responding to these symptoms with fear, and the avoidance and escape responses fire so automatically that patients may have little sense of what it is like to just sit and experience the sensations. When asked what was so bad about the induced sensations, some patients may say: "I don't know, I just needed it to stop." For these patients, the clinician may provide the following coaching:

> Notice your urge to try to escape from or otherwise try to hurry away the symptoms. And when you find yourself trying to somehow push the symptoms away or make them stop, I want you to instead do nothing. Pay attention to the symptoms, let yourself notice them and see if you can find anything tolerable about them. I want you to be able to see what it is like when you let the symptoms be there, and do your best to let yourself relax and let the symptoms stay.

(4) The patient's interpretations of their experiences are reviewed with an intent to enhance the perceived tolerability of the sensations. The learning from each exposure is used as a frame for the next symptom induction, with the clinician asking the patient to try to see if he or she can become even more comfortable (relaxed and nonavoidant) with the next symptoms induction.

(5) Repeat Steps 2 to 4. How many times are the symptoms induced? One answer is that it typically takes three to four with any specific induction procedure, but a better answer is that it depends on how both the clinician approaches the exposure and how the patient responds to it. Let's get to these factors.

5.5.2. Personalized Approach

We labeled these previous procedures as a *generic* way to conduct interoceptive exposure. The generic method relies on relatively passive learning of safety in response to repeated exposure, with the clinician providing a frame for what to do in response to the symptoms—relax with the symptoms, noticing what they feel like and that they can be experienced safely, if not, ultimately, relatively comfortably—without too much additional instruction. However, if exposure is the active learning of safety (it is!), specifically, the development of new associative and interpretative meaning of these symptoms, then anything that can hasten the salience and depth of these "safety" memories should be considered for use with interoceptive exposure.

One strategy for doing this is to make full use of the patient's previous learning of safety. This learning undoubtedly includes many of the sensations listed in Figure 5.2. For example, feelings of rapid heart rate, dyspnea, or nausea may have been felt in more intensive athletic encounters, and flushing and dizziness may have been induced as part any of a number of childhood games (e.g., spinning in a circle or rolling down a hill). The popularity and joyfulness of this last symptom induction—dizziness from spinning in a circle or rolling down a hill—provides an ideal emotional backdrop for re-establishing safety in response to these sensations. Indeed, even patients with substantial fears of dizziness currently, have had a history of joyfully experiencing these sensations in childhood. For these reasons, we most frequently initiate interoceptive exposure with *head rolling*:

There are at least three reasons to start exposure with head rolling:

(1) Patients often have fears of head rolling–induced dizziness/disorientation that are in the mild to moderate range, allowing for relatively quick adaptation to this stimulus without a wealth of overlearned escape responses. This is particularly relevant for the patient who expresses concerns about being able to tolerate interoceptive exposure and/or its effectiveness.
(2) The dizziness/disorientation from this procedure passes quickly, allowing for multiple brief trials of symptom induction to be completed.
(3) As noted, most patients have a childhood history of pleasurable interpretations of dizziness (e.g., induced by rolling down hills, spinning in a circle), allowing for the elicitation of positive memory associations to counteract the automatic fear interpretations of the dizziness/disorientation symptoms.

Hence, to speed the active learning of safety in response to feared sensations of dizziness, we routinely complement generic exposure experiences with recall of early positive experiences. For example, after initial interceptive exposure with head rolling (e.g., 2–3 initial exposures with review of symptoms induced, coaching, and responses to symptoms: Relative relaxation vs. urges to avoid/escape), we would discuss with the patient his or her own history of inducing dizziness as a child. In this discussion, contextual details are collected (what childhood friends were present, where was the spinning/rolling done, how did friends react, did they fall down in the grass). With this information collected, the clinician then uses these details to evoke a clear image (with friends, in a backyard, laughing and falling down, smell of grass in the summertime), and then head rolling exposure is completed again. During this symptom induction, the patient is asked to interpret the induced sensation in the context of these childhood memories. The change in response can be dramatic. Patients who in the initial exposure tensed up and braced their bodies against the induced dizziness, sometimes (i.e., in about a third of cases) ended the exposure with a broad smile on their faces. The same sensation that induced fear in the last exposure practice induced a smile when associated with the childhood memory. Figures 5.3 to 5.5 illustrates this process in terms of the memory node model presented in Chapter 2.

Figure 5.3 shows the association between dizziness and the patient's long-standing panic responses after initial rehearsals of doing nothing in response to these sensations. Figure 5.4 then depicts the recall and linking of dizziness with another well-formed and powerful memory from childhood. In this interpretive context, very different emotions are elicited (the childhood memory provided the interpretative context, rich in associative meaning to the dizziness). One or two more exposures are then completed in the context of childhood memories of dizziness to help set in this new association, with Figure 5.5 showing the

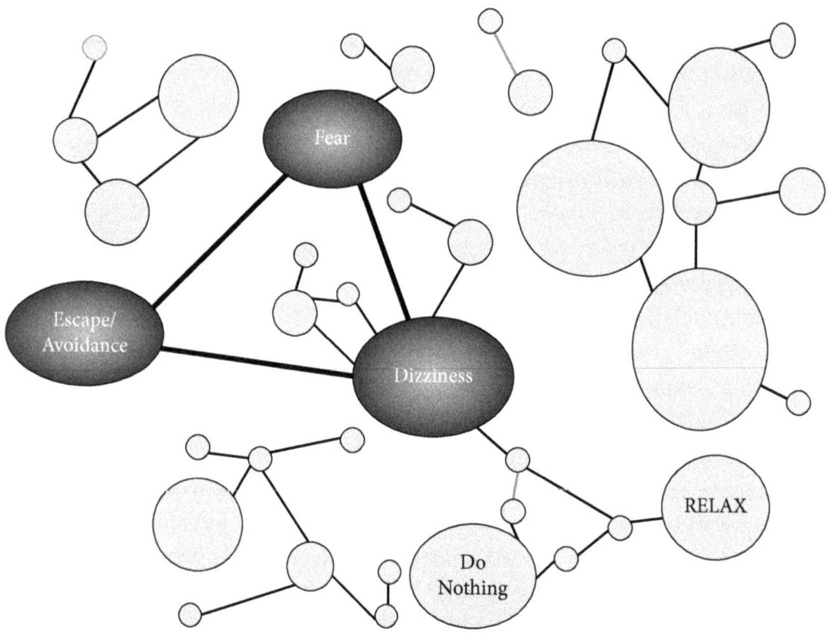

Figure 5.3 Memory association diagram (node model) showing the strong fear association of panic sensations to the observing nonresponse of doing nothing to manage the sensations and relaxing with them.

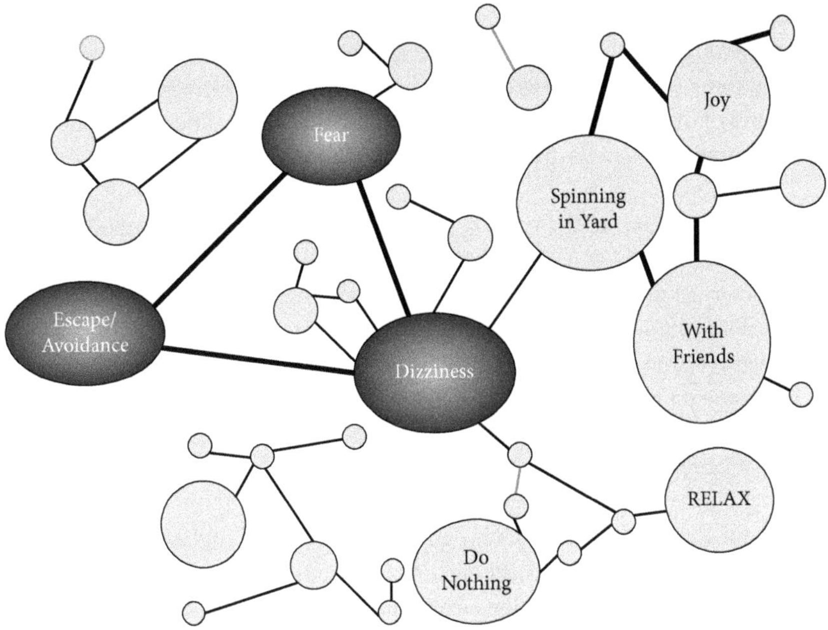

Figure 5.4 Memory association diagram (node model) showing the association of panic sensations to early memories of pleasure/safety.

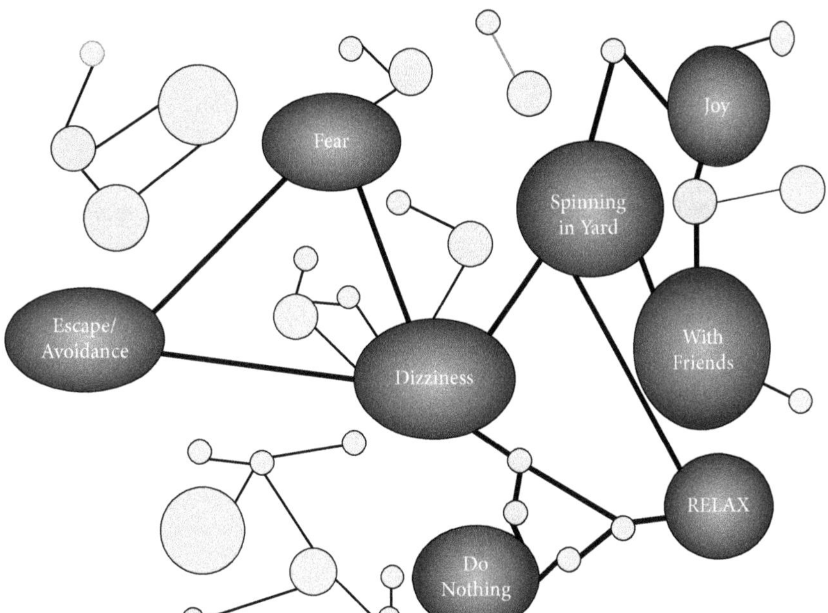

Figure 5.5 Memory association diagram (node model) showing the strengthening of the alternative (childhood) meaning of dizziness and the strengthening of the non-response to dizziness that is linked to this symptom meaning.

strengthening of the link to childhood memories and a relaxed nonresponse to symptoms (with these links competing with the fear interpretations of the symptom of dizziness. As the patient experiences her very different response to the symptoms of induced dizziness, the clinician may want to point out:

> This is the essence of the value of interoceptive exposure. The tolerability of symptoms, and, in fact, their entire meaning, is largely dependent on how you interpret them. You have just had some experiences where the exact same symptom (dizziness) is experienced as aversive or one of pleasure that can be enjoyed. The core of what we are going to do in this phase of treatment is to expand on this initial learning—to use a step-by-step process to eliminate fears of sensations and to make sure that these symptoms cannot evoke self-perpetuating patterns of anxiety, fear, and avoidance.

And for the rest of patients who do not end the head rolling exposure with a smile on their face, what is the next step? Almost exactly the same, because the recall of childhood inductions of dizziness may not push the experience all the way to joy, but it reliably reduces the aversiveness of the experience. Indeed, for patients with panic disorder or PTSD, it is important to underscore how they approached the *latter head rolling* exposures differently—being open to experiencing the sensation in a new way. Figure 5.6 is helpful to this process, to

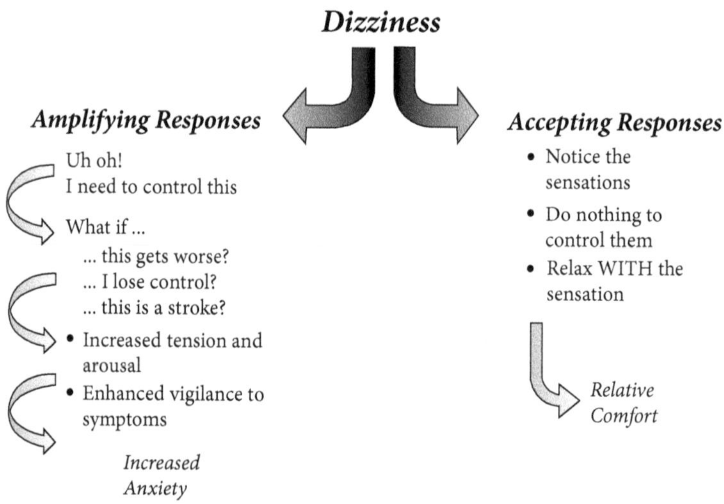

Figure 5.6 Retraining responses to symptom induction: amplifying and accepting responses. Figure adapted from Otto et al., *10-minute CBT,* Oxford, England: Oxford University Press, 2011, p. 67.

emphasize the amplification of symptoms that results from fear-of-fear cycles and the opposite reactions that characterizing accepting/relaxing with the induced sensations/emotions.

5.5.3. What Is the Patient to Do during Exposure?

Because of the way in which fearful reactions to anxiety/arousal symptoms further escalate symptoms (the core feature of fear-of-fear cycle), it is important to help patients feel the alternative to these responses. So far, we have used words like "pay attention to the symptoms, let yourself notice them, and see if you can find anything tolerable about them." The goal of this coaching is acceptance of symptoms—it is active rehearsal of nonresponse (i.e., to relax with the symptoms does not mean to reduce arousal, but to not try to control or protect against the symptoms)—to do less, not more, when confronted by the symptoms. If there is an active frame for this process, it is best described as *playful curiosity*, which describes an openness to experience the induced sensations in a new way, to turn one's attention toward and not away from these symptoms, and to examine afresh how dangerous, aversive, or intolerable these experiences are.

In this process, there is a similarity to mindfulness—of accepting experiential content without judgment. Yet, in contrast to traditional mindfulness training, interoceptive exposure ensures practice with acceptance and nonaction to sensations *under conditions of high emotional arousal.* That is, while mindfulness can be considered as "cool emotional acceptance training," interoceptive exposure offers "hot emotional acceptance training"—training that will not require later generalization from the quiet and supportive atmosphere of meditation training to the very different state of anxious arousal in a potential agoraphobia-inducing situation. All of this is important because the reaction to the symptoms determines the subsequent intensity of the symptoms: Fearful responses to fear increase fear. This is why programming an alternative response to symptoms is so important. A calm and accepting response to symptoms stops the fear-of-fear cycle.

5.5.4. Thinking about Interoceptive Exposure Broadly

Whenever maladaptive emotional avoidance is evident in a patient's functioning, there is a potential role for interceptive exposure. When Phillipe, a 52-year-old investment banker is reluctant to discuss issues with his ailing father (due to extreme discomfort with feelings of sadness or regret), there is a potential role for interoceptive exposure. When Anisa cannot hold a civil discussion with her daughter because she becomes overwhelmed by her own emotional experience, there is a role for interceptive exposure. And when Jake is having trouble controlling his use of alcohol when he is upset by the day-to-day challenges of his work and home life, there is a potential role for interoceptive exposure.

In sum, we would like clinicians to consider interoceptive exposure as a core tool for promoting emotional acceptance and tolerance whenever patients are having challenges with their own emotional or somatic experience. Said differently, emotional avoidance can frequently derail or slow the process of therapy. To reduce this avoidance, and to facilitate the ability to delve into emotional content, interoceptive exposure provides an essential tool. We also believe that enhanced emotional acceptance and tolerance is one of the general factors in therapy for the promotion of well-being and resilience. For patients with more extreme challenges in this domain (i.e., patients with panic disorder, PTSD, or other anxiety disorders), interoceptive exposure is an essential tool in therapy, leading patients from dramatic levels of fear and avoidance to greater tolerability and adaptability. Yet the endpoint is the same for these and other patients in therapy: To continue to apply lessons from interceptive exposure for greater well-being regardless of the context in which negative emotions and sensations arise.

For the targeted goal of treating a panic or anxiety-related disorder, or for additional treatment goals, it is important to think broadly about what sort of procedures can be used for interoceptive exposure. Table 5.2 listed those that are most relevant to panic-related concerns. But patients may have other patterns of intolerance of emotions that are not related to panic-like episodes. Table 5.3 lists some alternative procedures for directly targeting other emotions that may drive maladaptive avoidance or escape behaviors. Some of these maladaptive

Table 5.3 Example of Alternative Interoceptive Exposure Procedures

Emotion Targeted	Procedure
Fatigue	**Sleep deprivation:** Ask the patient to limit sleep to three hours the night before the session (no driving to the session)
Cigarette craving	**Withdrawal challenge:** As the patient to refrain from consuming cigarettes three hours before the session and two hours after the session
Boredom	**Wall staring:** Staring at a blank wall in the office while thinking, "I am so bored."
Sadness	**Movies:** Select from YouTube: Bambi's mother's death scene, death scene from *The Champ*, father scene from *Field of Dream*, etc. **Imagery:** Of a patient's personal sad memory

behaviors may include negative health behaviors that reflect coping motives such as smoking, drinking, or eating in response to negative affect. Maladaptive behaviors may also include procrastination behaviors that are also motivated by the desire to avoid the negative affect (guilt, anxiety, boredom) associated with other tasks, such as required work or school tasks. Accordingly, we would like clinicians to evaluate when interoceptive exposure can be used as a form of resilience training to help patients enhance their ability to accept and withstand the presence of a wide variety of avoided emotional experiences.

In addition to directly enhancing tolerance of emotions and related physical sensations, interoceptive exposure procedures also provide a context for learning alternative and adaptive responses to these emotional cues. Keep in mind that safety learning is an active learning process. Throughout this chapter, we describe the opposite of fearful and anxiogenic responses to symptoms as doing nothing to manage (and noticing and relaxing) with the symptoms. We think this core acceptance learning provides a substrate for additional adaptive responses. That is, once a fearful response to the emotional cues passes, individuals have the ability to choose adaptive responses to the situation at hand that are not driven by intensive escape motivations. This is a valuable skill for everyday functioning as well as treating an anxiety disorder. As such, we believe that, in addition to the core cessation of fear-of-fear cycles, the endpoint of therapy with interoceptive exposure is a patient who has:

- The ability to treat emotions as information—as a signal of the presence of a novel or historical cue that evokes this emotion. This emotional information may be accurate (a true signal) or inaccurate (a false alarm, for a current situation).
- With a greater capacity to tolerate emotional content, the ability to better analyze the significance (accuracy) of this information, thus facilitating decisions on how to act on the emotion.
- With greater capacity to tolerate emotional content, the ability to persist longer in emotional situations, opening up the possibility for greater problem-solving, conflict resolution, and goal attainment.

With these adaptive endpoints in mind, it is now time to consider issues and strategies for staging interoceptive exposure across sessions.

5.5.5. Progression

The pace and starting point for interoceptive exposure is a personalized decision between patient and clinician and can be titrated based on the tolerance of an individual patient. This section illustrates how to pace exposure for a patient with strong concerns about symptoms (e.g., who had difficulty with the lower-level sensations induced such as dizziness/disorientation). For this patient, we want to ensure that he or she has a well-developed cognitive map on how to respond to induced sensations before a broader program of interoceptive exposure is enacted. For this patient, the intensity of sensations can be downgraded until relative comfort with the symptoms is achieved. For the most challenging patients—those who have such an automatic fear response to even subtle sensations—we as clinicians may have to step away from feared sensations altogether to try to establish initial experiences with nonreactivity to somatic stimuli. For example, rather persisting with head rolling for a highly sensitized patient, we may shift to lightly tapping the leg with a pencil and rehearsing comfortable nonresponse to the mildly annoying (but otherwise comfortable) sensations of being repeatedly tapped on the leg. During the tapping, the clinician rehearses the same core acceptance elements: Noticing the sensations, evaluating them, and becoming as comfortable as possible without trying to hurrying them away. Once this skill is learned with the relatively comfortable sensation of tapping, then the clinician returns to a lower-level feared sensations, rehearsing reacting to the feared sensation in the same way as the tapping.

By way of metaphor, we think of this process as akin to making a path through tall grass during a hike. It is most challenging to make the initial path—it is easy to get lost and overwhelmed—but by repeatedly walking the path, the way to proceed gets more and more clear. Once the way to walk forward is clear, then regular exposure can progress session by session.

It is the clinician's job structure a stepwise process of increasing the intensity and degree of fearfulness of the induced sensations/emotions (e.g., progressing through the hierarchy toward the most feared sensations on the Sensitivity to Somatic and Emotional Experiences Survey (Table 5.1). In arranging the hierarchy, clinicians should keep in mind the duration of symptoms. As noted, we start with head rolling because recovery from the symptoms (dizziness/disorientation) happens quickly after head rolling is stopped. This gives the patient a nice sense of control while tolerability to the sensations is learned. In contrast, hyperventilation-induced dizziness, tingling, or numbness is a more intensely feared induction, and the symptoms last longer (e.g., 45 seconds) after the induction is completed. As such, clinicians introduce this exposure only after there is evidence that patients can tolerate longer-lasting symptoms, working up for truly long-lasting symptoms such as those from caffeine use (the coffee bean induction, which may give symptoms lasting longer than an hour). In addition to modulating the intensity and duration of symptoms, clinicians also need to consider the way in which contexts modify symptom meaning.

5.5.6. Attending to Context

For most people, the meaning of somatic sensations and emotions is situation dependent. Tearing up in a conversation with a valued friend has different meaning than tearing up when giving a speech. Likewise, having heart palpitations while in a theater has a different meaning than those same symptoms at home. The situational context modifies the availability of perceived help, escape, or embarrassment, and, as such, it modifies the catastrophic consequences anticipated with the symptoms. Clinicians who have treated many patients who fear panic and related bodily sensations have a natural sense of the idiosyncratic ways in which concerns over panic leads to unique patterns of avoidance. For example, are fears of anxiety symptoms greater while in public situations where escape behaviors are noticeable like grocery store, the hairdresser, or bank; or are they greater in a car when traveling far from home, where concerns about the inability to cope or impending death can dominate. Part of the value of the Sensitivity to Somatic and Emotional Experiences Survey (Table 5.1) is that it allows clinicians to map specific fears onto particular avoided situations in relation to anxiogenic interpretations of symptoms. The survey can thus offer guidance on when induced sensations will be harder to cope with.

The initial context for all interoceptive exposure exercises is the clinician's office, where the cycle of explanation, induction, and review of symptom meanings is generally repeated three to five times with any target symptom. The goal of in-session exposure practice is to have the patient experience an initial reduction in Subjective Units of Distress (SUDs) and positively experience leaning into fear as opposed to fighting it by engaging in safety behaviors. Daily homework will be prescribed as follows:

> Now the next step in the treatment is for you to practice this exposure at home and see if you can get bored by the resulting sensations. Specifically, I would like you to conduct three exposures at home each day, working across the week to get comfortable with higher and higher levels of symptoms. From our practice here today, you know the symptoms that you are going to induce, but they may strike you differently when you do it at home when I am not around. So, to give you some practice for what it feels like to do this at home alone, I am going to have you induce the symptoms one more time in here, while I step out of the

> office for a few minutes. I want you to notice whether you tell yourself anything differently, or whether you have a stronger urge to hurry the symptoms away when I am not sitting here with you. Remember that your goal is to become as comfortable as you can *with* the symptoms.

By stepping out of the office, the clinician gives the patient preliminary experience on how reactions to symptoms may change by context. When the clinician returns to the office, any difficulties with the symptoms in the "alone" context should be reviewed, and additional exposures or practice should be completed in session until the patient is comfortable with the "alone" procedure. Doing so meets a principle for exposure: Have the patient complete procedures successfully in session prior to assigning these symptom inductions in home practice.

The transition from in-session interoceptive exposure to home interoceptive exposure represents only the first example of the task of generalizing a sense of safety with the target sensations/emotions to new contexts. That is, after comfort is achieved with an identified sensation/emotion in session and at home, the next step is to practice interoceptive exposure in feared situations. To provide an example, let's consider the case of Anna who has particular fear of dizziness sensations in public and while driving. Anna's Sensitivity to Somatic and Emotional Experiences Survey reflects these concerns as is evident in Table 5.4.

Discussion with Anna reveals that symptoms while driving are much more concerning than symptoms in a store, so interoceptive exposure practice in a store is collaboratively selected as a reasonable next step from home practice. Depending on how threatening this next step is, the clinician may select an interim step of practicing the head rolling interoceptive exposure in a store nearby the clinician's office. For example, after reviving the sense of comfort with head rolling–induced symptoms during a repeat exposure in the office, the clinician and patient may walk to a nearby business (a coffee shop, bookstore, or convenience store), walk to the back, and induce head rolling symptoms while holding on to a shelf. Once the symptoms are induced, the patient buys a small item or interacts briefly with the clerk before leaving the store and meeting the clinician outside. Results are discussed and, depending on comfort level, the interoceptive exposure can be repeated in the store, or the clinician can go ahead and assigned independent practice for the client. The next week, the clinician may repeat this same process with head rolling practices in the car according to the following schedule:

(1) Head rolling while seated in a parked car at home.
(2) Head rolling in a parked car away from home.
(3) Head rolling and then driving the car from a parked location to home.

Table 5.4 Anna's Completed Sensitivity to Somatic and Emotional Experiences Survey

Sensation or Emotion	Applicable	Example of Related Avoidance	Anticipated Threat	Rank Order
Feeling dizzy or lightheaded	√	I never drive when I feel at all dizzy	Losing control and crashing the car	3
Rapid or irregular heartbeat				
Dyspnea	√	Call my husband or best friend; leave public places	I might suffocate or fain t from not enough air	2
Chest pain or pressure	√	I just hate it	If it gets worse, it may be a heart attack	5
Numbness and Tingling (face, scalp, or extremities)	√	I flee home if this happens	I don't want to lose control in public, especially if this is a stroke	1
Face flushing				
Sweating	√	I go home	I don't want people to think something is wrong with me	
Trembling				
Upset stomach, nausea				
Derealization or depersonalization	✓	I leave stores to be alone, I never drive when I feel this	People will think I am crazy; I may lose control	4
Sadness		I hate it	I act happy; I should not be sad	
Boredom		I wish . . . I am too nervous to be bored		
Guilt				

Table 5.5 illustrates a generic ordering of interoceptive exposure over units of time. In the figure, the units of time (1–8) could be sessions or parts of sessions, depending on how fast the patient gets comfortable with the targeted interoceptive exposure-induced sensations and emotions.

When considering the influence of contexts on the meaning of interoceptive cues, it is important to also consider internal contexts. Doing interoceptive exposure when rested is very different than doing interoceptive exposure when fatigued. Likewise, doing interoceptive exposure when feeling supported at home can be very different from doing interoceptive exposure after a difficult argument with one's spouse. In these examples, the contexts bias the interoceptive exposure in terms of threat interpretations. Using the memory node model (see Figure 5.7), the right panel as compared to the left panel illustrates the relative difficulty of learning safety when conducting interoceptive exposure in a context denoting threat.

After progressing through interoceptive exposure exercise across relevant symptom types, symptom intensities, and situation al contexts, it may be time for the clinician to then ensure that interoceptive exposure is conducted across threatening and nonthreatening contexts (e.g., when rested and when fatigued, when supported and when interpersonally vulnerable, on good days and bad

Table 5.5 Example of the Pacing of Exposure across Situations and across Intensities of Induced Sensations

	Situational Context			
Sensation Intensity	**In Office**	**At Home**	**Lower Situational Discomfort**	**High Situational Discomfort**
Mild/moderate interoceptive exposure intensity Method 1	1	1	3	5
Moderate/high interoceptive exposure intensity Method 1	2	2	4	5
Mild/moderate interoceptive exposure intensity Method 2	2	3	4	5
Moderate/high interoceptive exposure intensity Method 2	3	4	5	6
Mild/Moderate interoceptive exposure intensity Method 3	4	5	6	7
Moderate/high interoceptive exposure intensity Method 3	5	6	7	8

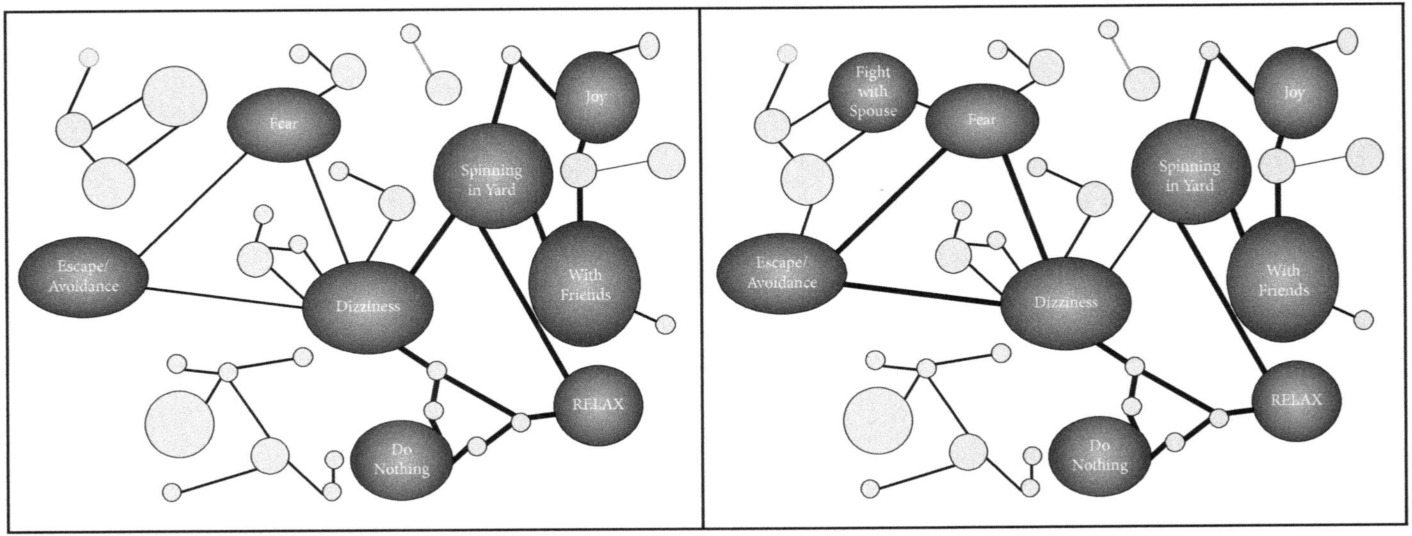

Figure 5.7 Memory association diagram (node model) showing the potential effects of a threatening context on safety learning to dizziness.

days, etc.). Life usually arranges these varying contexts, and hence it is up to the clinician to monitor whether exposure is being skipped in particular emotional/vulnerability contexts. If so, additional care needs to be taken to assign interoceptive exposure practice specifically when these contexts arise. Alternatively, clinicians can use imagery more at vulnerable times (e.g., as per Chapter 7) and conduct interoceptive exposure after these context inductions (e.g., imagining when one last felt interpersonally vulnerable after relationship conflict).

Finally, contextual manipulations can also include the internal context due to what the patient is saying to himself or herself (i.e., thought content). For example, heart palpitations can be experienced very differently in the clinician's office versus when one is on his or her own with the thought "I think this is a heart attack; I may die." At some point, the clinician may wish to reintroduce specific thoughts to be the backdrop for interoceptive exposure. This is not as aversive as it may seem. In our clinics, we have done this by having either the clinician repeat the fearsome thought over and over again during the interoceptive exposure or, in group settings, have the patients pair up and say the fearsome thoughts to each other. The most common response to these procedures, when properly introduced, is laughter. The patients get experience with interoceptive exposure in the context of catastrophic thoughts and have an opportunity to experience these thoughts with a very different affect.

5.5.7. Attending to Safety Behaviors

As noted in Chapter 2, safety behaviors—the avoidance and escape maneuvers that the patient uses to manage his or her fears—can nullify safety learning (e.g., "The feared outcome would have happened had I not had my water with me, had my antacids with me, had my cell phone so I can call my spouse, stood near the exit sign, stood near my friend, etc."). In treatment, we do not want our patient's sense of safety to be conditional, that is, dependent on whether escape or avoidance with a safety behavior is available. For fuller learning of safety, safety behaviors should be faded from interoceptive exposure practice over time. For example, the clinician may start a discussion on safety behaviors as follows:

> You have been doing well so far getting used to some of the sensations that have bothered you. As you know, you first got used to these sensations here in session with me, and then we sent you home to work to become bored with these sensations when you are home alone. We then transitioned to helping you get bored with some of these sensations when sitting in your car or when you are in a store. Now we are going to start to work on helping you feel comfortable with

these sensations when you don't have some of your safety strategies with you. For example, you mentioned that you always carry your cell phone with you so you can call your husband or a friend, and you almost always have water with you so you can use the feel of cool water to try to calm down. Our next step is to help you know that you can be fine with sensations, even if you don't have cool water and even if you can't make a call. Does the importance of this sort of practice make sense to you?"

Of safety behaviors, medication use is a prominent feature. Interoceptive exposure while on medications does not necessarily generalize to interoceptive exposure off medication. Likewise, interoceptive exposure while carrying medication (e.g., an "emergency" benzodiazepine) does not necessarily generalize to interoceptive exposure without carrying emergency medication. Because of the importance of medication contexts, we have devoted Chapter 8 to medication issues in exposure therapy. At this point though, it is useful to think of safety behavior elimination and specific anxiogenic thought exposures as elements that may need to be added to the "high situational discomfort" column in the following Exposure Planning Worksheet (see Box 5.1) to ensure full safety learning to the targeted sensations. The worksheet is used to make sure that a patient's particular feared cues and contexts are taken into account in exposure planning. This checklist can be populated, in part, from the patient's Sensitivity to Somatic and Emotional Experiences Survey (as well as measures such as the Panic Appraisal Inventory and ASI; see Chapter 9), but offers a broader framework for the staging of interoceptive exposure in more threatening contexts.

5.6. Use of Naturalistic Symptom Evocation and Extending Treatment Gains

Interoceptive exposure uses a range of exercises to induce symptoms that are close to those experienced during anxiety and panic. Yet, not all patients can generalize from these explicitly induced sensations to those that arise naturally from emotional/phobic experiences. Accordingly, it is useful to plan for these difficulties by including more naturalistic symptom evocations in treatment. That is, rather than assigning interoceptive exposure, clinicians can assign entry into an avoided situation, treating the anticipatory or in-situation anxiety as if it were induced by interoceptive exposure. Specifically, the patient is to plan for what symptoms may arise, cue the symptoms by going into a feared situation, pay attention to the exact symptoms induced, and rehearse the "doing nothing" response. If symptoms dissipate particularly quickly, patients can use interoceptive

Box 5.1 Interoceptive Exposure Planning Worksheet

Patient: *Anna* **Date:** *8-12-2018*

Target threat appraisals (use response from the Sensitivity to Somatic and Emotional Experiences Survey):

Feared symptom: *being perceived as incompetent* Rating: 70%

Feared symptom: Rating:

Feared symptom: Rating:

Feared symptom: Rating:

Goals

Produce moderate symptoms using visual zing strategies (staring at heater vent, staring at hand) and doing nothing to manage the symptoms.

Aggravating Contexts (contexts in which the fear of emotions/symptoms is worse)

- ❑ Time of day:
- ❑ Locations:
- ❑ Presence of others:
- ❑ Fatigue or background emotion(s):
- ❑ Specific thoughts:
- ❑ Duration of symptoms:
- ❑ Other cue(s):
- ❑ Other cue(s):

Safety Behaviors (plan when to fade/eliminate)

- ❑ Contact with others: *cell phone contact with husband, friend*
- ❑ Food/drink: *bottle of water*
- ❑ Medications:
- ❑ Cognitive rituals/lucky sayings (list): *"I will be OK."*
- ❑ Social errors/mishaps (specify):
- ❑ Body posture (e.g., sitting leaning against a wall)

Set specific and achievable behavioral goal (based on goals and manipulations above):

Start with three interoceptive exposure inductions in the office, conduct a fourth with the therapist out of the room, conduct a fifth with the patient's phone and water bottle removed.

exposure to bring back select sensations and again rehearse doing nothing in response to these symptoms. The following excerpt exemplifies this approach:

> For the last few weeks we have been having you use interoceptive exposure to create and practice accepting symptoms in some of your feared situations. And it has been going well—you told me today about how well you did with dizziness induced in your car. For practice this week, I would like you to start skipping the "middleman." That is, I want you to see if you can evoke symptoms by going into specific situations that used to bother you. For example, I remember that you told me that you really get anxious around heights. I wonder if you can use this concern about heights as an interoceptive exposure procedure. For example, you may want to park on the higher level of the parking structure down the street and then walk to the barrier and look down. When you look down, you are likely to get the symptoms you mentioned (dizziness and that sinking feeling in your stomach). You can treat that like the feelings you get from head rolling, but induce it by safely standing at the waist-high barrier. Your goal is to react to it the same way you reacted to the sensations you induced in your car: Pay attention to the symptoms, notice exactly what they feel like, and see how well you can relax and feel comfortable with the symptoms present. How does that sound—using heights instead of head rolling to induce and get further comfortable with these symptoms?

A further strategy for therapeutic use of naturalistic symptom evocations is to attend to emotions and symptoms arising from interpersonal challenges. We think of this as explicit practice extending the benefit of in-session interoceptive exposure exercises to promote emotional tolerance/acceptance skills in relation to important values and life areas where they are relevant. One area for practice concerns interpersonal challenges. Problems and conflicts with people drive many of our negative emotions (e.g., anxiety, sadness, guilt, frustration). Listed in Box 5.2 are some common situations where negative emotions may be evoked. Again, the goal is to respond to the sensations that arise from these experiences exactly as one would in an in-session or at-home interoceptive exposure practice. Rather than having to induce these sensations with head rolling or hyperventilation, the goal is to let everyday interpersonal challenges do it for the patient. Practice of this skill is aided by the following monitoring form. On the form, the patient is to record not only what symptoms were evoked by these interpersonal situations, but also how the symptoms were experienced differently once the symptoms were treated as if evoked in an interoceptive exposure practice.

Table 5.6 Prototypical Session Content

Task	Activities	Time
1. Agenda setting	• Discuss session goals • Determine session activities	5 min.
2. Assessment	• Review symptom severity • Review what has been learned from the last session	5 min.
3. Review of homework	• Review interoceptive exposure experiences and symptom interpretations • Decide on relevant interoceptive exposure practice for the current session	5 min.
4. Practice	• Preparation for symptoms to be experienced • interoceptive exposure induction (noticing and not avoidance induced symptoms • Review of symptom interpretation • Repeat	30 min.
5. Review and homework assignment	• Review what has been learned • Discuss how learning can be applied • Discuss the nature of home practice	5-10 min.

5.7. Targeting Fears of Emotions and Related Bodily Sensations across the Disorders

Targeting fears of somatic arousal is central to panic disorder, but it also has applications for other anxiety and phobic disorders whenever there is substantial fear or avoidance of emotions and related sensations. As previously noted, these fears are particularly high in panic disorder and PTSD but are also elevated across the rest of the anxiety disorders.

In the application of interoceptive exposure to PTSD, the goal is to remove the ability of anxiety/panic to automatically trigger trauma memories. That is, in PTSD it is as if the trauma memory has co-opted the meaning of anxiety/fear so that the experience of anxiety itself becomes a trauma cue. Under these conditions, exposure is particularly challenging because exposure evokes anxiety and anxiety may evoke further trauma memories, leading to a feed-forward cycle of fear-of-fear that is caught up in the fear of trauma memories.

Interoceptive exposure provides a way to "pretreat" the fears associated with anxiety symptoms themselves so that anxiety becomes a tolerable experience

Box 5.2 Values-Based Naturalistic Exposure Checklist

Instructions: Listed below are some common situations where negative emotions may be evoked; the goal is to be aware of these situations and to use them to rehearse the "be aware of symptoms and relax with them" response that is an essential part of promoting emotional resilience. The goal is to respond to the sensations that arise from the following experiences exactly as one would in an in-session or at-home interoceptive exposure practice. Record not only what symptoms were evoked by these interpersonal situations, but also how the symptoms were experienced differently once they were treated as if evoked in an interoceptive exposure practice.

Situation	Emotions and sensations evoked by the situation	When approaching these sensations like interoceptive exposure, how did your behavior change?
Conflict with a romantic partner		
Handling a work-related conflict		
Disciplining children when frustrated		
Managing interactions with a difficult mother-in-law		
Thinking about completing a project for which you are late		
Thinking about a disappointment/failure		
Other		

rather than a cue for trauma memories. To aid with this process, patients may need explicit help remembering anxiety and fear episodes before the onset of PTSD, and rehearsal that PTSD does not "get to own" every experience of anxiety. Interoceptive exposure would proceed along the lines of what has been previously detailed, but the core discrimination between trauma memories and safety memories is different, as exemplified in Figure 5.8.

Used as a pretreatment for PTSD, interoceptive exposure sessions would be conducted for one to four sessions to ensure to promote relative comfort with the anxiety that will be elicited by imaginal exposures to trauma cues (Chapter 7).

The value of pretreatment with interoceptive exposures also is evident for obsessive-compulsive (O-C) and other disorders where exposure or exposure plus response prevention (ERP) is used to replace maladaptive responses to anxiety (Chapter 7). Interestingly, the use of interoceptive exposure for O-C related disorders is rarely discussed in the clinical research literature. Instead, there is emphasis on more situational cue exposure in an ERP format where an anxiety response is cued by exposure (e.g., touching feared objects for those with handwashing compulsions, listening to forbidden words for those with scrupulosity compulsions, leaving the house within several minutes for those with stove-checking compulsions, discarding "special" objects for those with hoarding compulsions), and compulsive responses (designed to neutralize the perceived threat) are blocked. Completing any of these exposures may evoke a

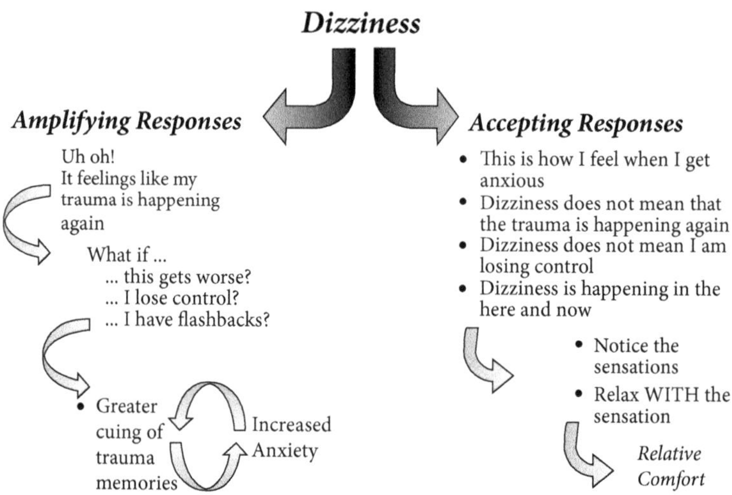

Figure 5.8 Retraining responses to symptom induction: amplifying and accepting responses for posttraumatic stress disorder.

strong anxiety response in patients, and indeed, most patients are able to learn that this anxiety response is a false alarm, and the magnitude of the alarm (anxiety) dissipates over time. Yet, there are many patients who have such an anxiety response that engagement in ERP may be slowed or avoided due to an inability to tolerate the anxiety. For these patients, we consider whether an initial interoceptive exposure treatment phase (targeting enhancing comfort with the anxiety signal) may make progress through situational exposures that much more bearable. As with our earlier example of snake phobia, interoceptive exposure would be used to parse the O-C exposure to two parts: Exposure to the anxiety and then exposure to the cue for the compulsion (with response prevention).

With this approach, the clinician would prepare the patient for typical O-C exposures by first conducting several sessions of interoceptive exposure, helping the patient to treat the anxiety signal as a false alarm by directly targeting these symptoms outside the context of O-C ERP exercises. Interoceptive exposure would be used as prelearning to help the patient develop the ability to better "do nothing in response to anxiety or other symptoms" well before the patient is introduced to the sudden provocation of these symptom as part of the ERP procedure. This sort of prelearning is not much different from selecting a lower-level stimulus for exposure (e.g., a less "contaminated" object for ERP for a patient with a handwashing compulsion), allowing the patient to "learn the ropes" with the ERP similar to the way we recommend patients "learn the ropes" with interoceptive exposure with head rolling. However, there is an important difference: Rather than being simply a lower-level stimulus on a hierarchy, it is a cue in a different domain—internal versus external—and hence represents a different type of preparatory learning.

In sum, interoceptive exposure holds particular value for any patient who is progressing slowly in a situational or imaginal exposure paradigms due to concerns about his or her ability to tolerate resulting symptoms. In short, because anxiety may escalate rapidly during these exposures, pretreatment of fears of symptoms holds the promise for greater comfort during situational or imaginal exposures and helps the patient attend more directly to the disconfirmation of contamination fears (rather than focusing on the desire to escape the induced anxiety).

5.8. Considering the Prototypical Session and Intervention

To review, the general theme of each session of exposure targeting the fears of emotions and related bodily sensations is to:

(1) Prepare patients for the sensations that are about to be induced, with prerehearsal of doing nothing to manage these sensations (to "relax" with the sensations).
(2) Induce the sensations.
(3) In the context of the sensations, rehearse acceptance and nonavoidant responses while paying attention to the actual sensations induced.
(4) Review what was learned from the exposure.
(5) Repeat in session several times.
(6) Assign home practice, ensuring that enough elements of home practice have been rehearsed so that success with the exposure is likely.

The type, intensity, and context for each interoceptive exposure to be rehearsed in and out of session is selected in relation to the patient's specific fear profile (your case formulation of core elements of his or her fears) as elucidated by the patient's Sensitivity to Somatic and Emotional Experiences Survey and/or the Exposure Planning Checklist. Clinicians should enter each session with a specific learning target in mind: "If today's session is successful, I want the patient to leave having learned that . . ." As always, the exposure session occurs in the context of collaborative planning of session content with the patient and may include the elements outlined in Table 5.6. In our experience, of all the exposure exercises, head rolling is most valuable for introducing interoceptive exposure, and hyperventilation is most generically valuable for extending initial gains.

Sessions with this format are repeated with the step-by-step approach of establishing initial safety to lower-order feared cues, ensuring that acceptance responses to these cues are well rehearsed and then increasing both the intensity and variety of interoceptive cues targeted in exposure. When safety to these cues is reached, then the exposure sessions emphasize expanding the context in which these cues are interpreted as safe. This process involves the elimination of safety behaviors as well as adding in contextual factors associated with threat (e.g., fatigue, interpersonal threat, phobic situations). In the latter stages of treatment, more naturalistic exposure procedures are emphasized, and there is a transition to additional value-based exposures to meet the goal of promoting emotional tolerance and acceptance more generally. In this final phase, the clinician plays a role not only as a force to reduce psychopathology, but also as a force to promote well-being across a wider range of emotional and situational cues that can be challenging for everyone. These core phases are depicted in Table 5.7.

Table 5.7 Phases of Treatment as Applied to Anxiety, Obsessional, and Trauma Disorders Characterized by Fears of Emotional and Related Somatic Sensations

Phase of Treatment	Aims	Activities
1	• Develop and refine case formulation • Socialize patient to interoceptive exposure using head rolling or other lower level interoceptive exposure • Experience initial success with exposure practice	• Assessment • Rehearsal of non-response to interoceptive exposure
2	• Learning to "do nothing to manage symptoms" in the context of additional interoceptive exposure exercises under varying intensities	• Diversify interoceptive exposure practices • Increase home interoceptive exposure
3	• Learning that safety is unconditional	• Expand learned safety to more contexts • Attend to safety behavior fading • Conduct relevant situational or imaginal exposure
4	• Promote emotional tolerance more generally	• Utilize naturalistic and additional emotional cues in exposure

5.9. Troubleshooting Some Nonresponse Traps

In the following paragraphs, we illustrate some of the common challenges encountered targeting the fears of emotions and related bodily sensations. For each subtype of challenges, we then provide compensatory behavior to help the patient respond more adaptively to feared sensations and emotions.

- *But I induced these sensations!* At times, patients may discount the safety learned to sensations induced in session, citing that these sensations are induced and the others "come out of the blue." For this response, we recommend starting a discussion about the similarity between the induced sensations and anxiety responses occurring away from therapy. Typically, a patient will state that he or she are highly similar in sensations but are wholly different "because I know I induced these." The clinician should then reflect, "So you are saying that the sensations are very similar in how they feel, but that the ones you induce in here are comfortable simply because you know you induced them." After the patient underscores this fact with a hearty "Yes," then the clinician should continue: "This is incredibly important to know, because you are saying that the difference between a panic response and a nonpanic response is simply due to what you say about the symptoms. If you say, 'I know where this comes from,' you don't panic." After the patient again says, more wistfully, "Yes," the clinician then continues, "So if we can bottle this 'I know where this comes from' response, you might become panic free." After the patient responds, "Potentially," the clinician recommends the following therapeutic tasks: Ask the patient to (a) play with the notion that he or she does or does not know the source of symptoms during the next exposure (e.g., "I don't know why this is happening now" vs. "Something must have upset me or cued my heart to beat fast"), (b) look for contextual cues that may explain initial symptoms occurring naturally and understand subsequent symptoms in the context of "I have panic disorder," and (c) work to generalize the calm response from "I know why this is happening" into out-of-session anxiety episodes.

- *I am not afraid of that!* At times, patients may display avoidance of sensations while reporting no fear of the sensations (an "I just don't like that" response). For these patients, it can be useful to spend time having them identify any differences they can identify in how they react to phobia-related and phobia-unrelated cues. For example, a clinician may sequentially have the patient examine his or her response to leg tapping and then to hyperventilation, then to leg tapping, and then again to hyperventilation again to help him or her identify subtle ways in which he or she may be engaging in "control" responses to the latter sensations. Effort is then devoted to helping the patient train up adaptive responses to the phobic cues, using the responses to leg tapping as a model. After a number of these rehearsals, the clinician might continue:

> Regardless of your level of fear to these sensations, I want to make sure that you are not pushed around by these sensations. Specifically, I want to ensure that you are able to get your work done, make good decisions, and feel as comfortable as you can *with* these sensations. To do that, we are going to start a process of exposure in more public situations where you have a goal (e.g., buy a coffee, talk to a clerk). The idea is to help rehearse doing this comfortably with the symptoms present.

This approach is consistent with both the goal of ensuring adaptive functioning as the core response to the once-phobic cue and to evaluate whether fears may be context dependent. By mixing symptoms across contexts, the patient will be completing an effective evaluation of moderators of potential fear while also achieving strong functioning across these situations.

- *Not if I don't say so!* There is a subtype of panic disorder that is not defined by a particular fear of any one symptom, but by a fear of unscripted emotional experience. Based on belief that one should be in control of one's emotions at all times, even subtle experience of emotion set off a panic-laden cycle to try to stifle, subvert, or otherwise control the emotion. In our less than thoughtful moments, we have termed this subtype "men's disease" due to its linkage to traditional male stereotypes of controlled emotionality. For this subtype of panic, we recommend a broad range of emotional exposure experiences, including the provocations exercises in Table 5.2. Coaching during the exposure includes discussion that emotions are reactive to the environment and that control comes from being comfortable with the emotional experience rather than stopping or otherwise inhibiting it. In monitoring of outcome of these exposures, we recommend monitoring the quality of interpersonal interactions. With less need to control the emotions induced by these interactions (sometimes by angrily terminating the conversation), the quality of the interpersonal interactions frequently increases.
- *Avoidance of sessions or of home practice.* The first response to avoided home practice is a functional analysis of how the homework felt in the home context. Our expectation is that home practice may be unexpectedly more threatening than what was practiced in session. If this is true, we can bridge the gap between in-session and out-of-session exposure. We have already exemplified one strategy for doing this—have the patient prepractice all homework assignments while the clinician briefly steps out of the office. Another alternative is to make all home exposure assignments clearly less challenging than the in-session practice, so that in-session confidence can help drive out-of-session practice on less threatening exposure items. Also, embarrassment about having to practice such exercises ("Having to do these stupid exercises says I am flawed or weak") can impair willingness to conduct home exposures.

5.10. Conclusions

In this chapter, we have applied the approach to preparing, implementing, and processing exposure therapy (as described generally in Chapter 3) to the fear of emotions and related physical sensations. We described general strategies as well as some of the variations on the core themes that are appropriate with patients with particularly pronounced fears of emotions/symptoms. Emphasis was placed on the active learning of a safety response to anxiety itself. This ability—to relax with the experience of anxiety—is important for resilience to a wide range of stressors. Accordingly, interoceptive exposure procedures are a tool for reducing anxiety and panic as well as promoting emotional tolerance and well-being. Indeed, learning to react differently to anxiety itself is such an important process, you will see ways in which interoceptive exposure is incorporated into the treatment of other fears in each of the next several chapters.

6
Fear of People

6.1. The Case of Sydney

Sydney is an African American female who comes to therapy because she feels lonely. At 38, she finds herself concerned about fulfilling her dream of having a family. She wants to be in a relationship, get married, and have children, yet is terrified of dating. Sydney characterizes the few dates she has had over the past decade as miserable. After several days of near-constant worry, she experiences several panic attacks in the hours leading up to a date, feels flustered and unable to be in the moment when she is on a date, and then has trouble not constantly thinking about what went wrong in the days that follow. Dating represents the top of the hierarchy of situations Sydney fears and avoids. Across several interpersonal (e.g., attending meetings at work, having lunch with colleagues, going to a party, etc.) and performance (e.g., giving a presentation, speaking up at a meeting, etc.) settings, she holds back because she is concerned about performing poorly and that such poor performance has negative consequences. Sydney's responses on the Appraisal of Social Concerns (ASC) questionnaire make clear that she expects to appear anxious (e.g., blushing, sweating, being tense) and that as a result others do not approve of her (e.g., reject her, laugh at her, ridicule her). In an attempt to manage these concerns, Sydney has adopted a repertoire of safety behaviors—her score on the Subtle Avoidance Frequency Examination (SAFE) was 73 (see Chapter 9 for a description of the measures). Specifically, she hardly goes into a situation without preparing (e.g., rehearses sentences in mind, grooms meticulously, wears make-up to hide blushing) and has made a habit of avoiding "risks" in social situations (e.g., avoids asking questions, speaks in short sentences, avoids eye contact).

Sydney thinks that she is so sensitive to rejection because her mom was always very critical of her growing up. She recounts a number of events—parties, school plays, sporting events—where her mom scolded her in front of her peers. Entering high school insecure and guarded as a result, Sydney had a hard time making new friends and often found herself the subject of mockery and discrimination. These negative experiences were particularly evident to her in performance situations in the predominately White high school she attended. Although she has been able to form meaningful intimate relationships, her two long-term romantic relationships ended because she claims she was too "possessive" of her boyfriends and uncomfortable and unwilling to socialize as a couple. Bright and ambitious, Sydney was an A+ student who majored in accounting in college. After receiving her master of business administration, she rose the ranks in a top accounting firm. Her peers and clients describe her as "perfect," someone who always delivers. Sydney finds this ironic, as she believes she underperforms, and although she has been able to achieve many of her career goals, she feels like she would achieve more if she was more assertive and more engaged in leadership activities. Her perfectionistic tendencies and concerns about others' perceptions have also affected her self-views. Sydney points to several flaws in her physical appearance (e.g., nose that is too big, lips that are too thin). She spends more time checking herself in the mirror than she considers reasonable and is planning on having corrective surgery in the next year. These body image concerns amplify her fears of dating and further increase her symptoms of depression. Sydney wants to feel more positive about herself, care less about what others think of her, and expand her social life from the occasional get-togethers with a few girlfriends, her twin sister, or her brother.

6.1.1. Making Sense of Why Sydney Feels the Way She Feels

Not everyone can point to specific experiences as being critical to the onset of their fears. And, there is no one-to-one relationship between negative childhood experiences and social anxiety disorder. Indeed, many who were the subject of criticism growing up do not fear people as adults, and in fact, some who were indicate these experiences were formative, helping them feeling more prepared to face the challenges later on in life. For Sydney, though, the criticism she received from her mother and peers shaped the belief that being liked by others takes hard work, especially for her. She believes her presence draws attention and negative evaluation from others because it communicates inferiority; being genuine is not an option for her. Instead, Sydney puts in considerable effort to either hide her perceived weaknesses or avoid people altogether. What's especially difficult for her is that many of these safety behaviors have paradoxical effects. That is, rather than feeling more at ease going into situations, Sydney's preparation routine and vigilance while being around others sends a powerful signal that something is wrong, which increases symptoms of anxiety, which, in turn, hamper her performance and reinforce this negative anxiety cycle (see Figure 6.1). This is no different from the patient with a dog phobia who makes sure that he brings a stick before he walks through the park on his way to work. Of course, grabbing the stick *feels* like the right thing to do when you believe that a vicious dog attack is probable, but doing so inadvertently turns up the steam, getting the alarm system activated in preparation to fight ("It's going to happen, and I better be

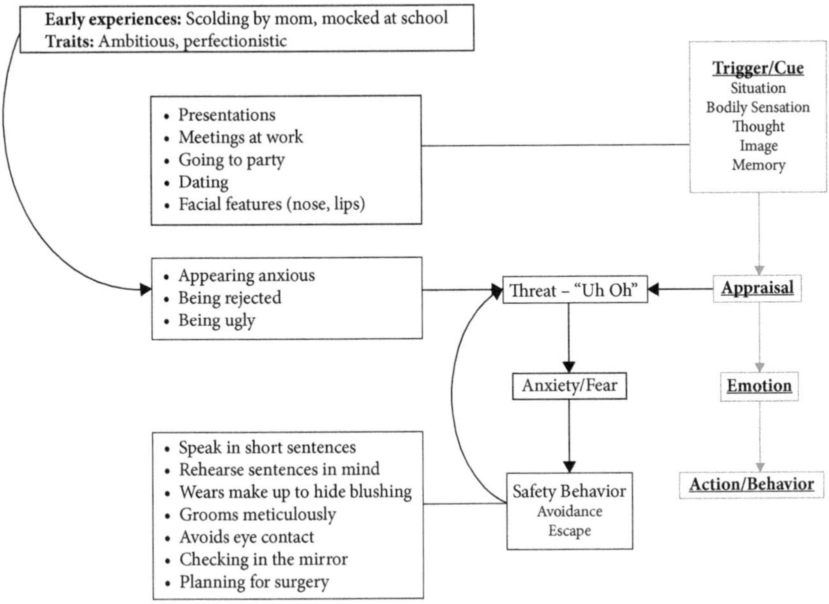

Figure 6.1 Sydney's initial case formulation.

ready"), and the result is an experience in the park that feels even more like being in a battle zone.

6.1.1.1. Trap 1: Judging False Alarms as True Alarms

The themes that Sydney describes are not foreign to us. Most of us desire being liked and prefer doing well in social interaction and performance situations. On top of that, we can all point to experiences where a good performance paid off, like a phone call that led to a job interview and the job interview that helped us land the job. And (social) media messages as well as conversations at work and social gatherings often convey that physical appearance contributes to success and satisfaction in life. The extent to which we as clinicians in our own life place significance on social competence and appearance can easily (mis)guide us in our case formulation and treatment planning. For example, we treated a 25-year-old single male who complained about the time he spent and the distress he experienced thinking about and checking his physical appearance. He added that he had consulted with a doctor who had prescribed a medication to delay hair loss. During supervision, the clinician indicated she believed this intervention was sensible as she agreed that balding at age 25 is something that should be prevented if possible. The clinician's view seemed reasonable to many, although not all other clinicians in the supervision group. Interestingly, though, all trainees uniformly agreed that enhancing his self-esteem by getting calf implants would be a bad idea. This example nicely illustrates that the clinician's own preferences or thinking style can influence one's ability to effectively identify targets for intervention. Certainly, the clinician's role is not to serve as an aesthetician in these situations as there are obviously no guidelines for useful enhancement. Instead, it's our job to help the patient determine whether an action—in this case, enhancement—serves as a safety behavior that maintains the fear cycle (i.e., enhancement functions to prevent a feared outcome) or whether it is a form of positive coping (i.e., enhancement functions to improve quality of life but is not selected to avert a feared outcome). When it's deemed a safety behavior, we encourage the patient to make it a target of intervention.

Obviously, recognizing the themes that fuel the negative emotions that bring patients to our practice can serve us well as it puts us in a better position to develop strong therapeutic relationships. When you find yourself nodding when your patient convincingly argues his fears are sensible, you're showing the first signs of falling into the trap of treating false alarms as true alarms. And this trap is not specific to the fear of people. Too often do we hear clinicians state, for example, that a patient's depression makes sense (and therefore imply, to some patients, that it is not amenable to treatment) because they would feel exactly the same if they faced the patient's current situation. So, how can we prevent ourselves from falling into that trap? It starts with recognition and self-monitoring. Let's go back to the case of Sydney. When you notice having difficulty finding fault with Sydney's approach to work and social situations, consider that a flag guiding you to be careful in your assessment. If Sydney has it right, why is it that her twin sister Keisha, who has nearly identical physical attributes and had similar experiences growing up, does not experience social anxiety or is overly occupied with perfecting her performance and physical appearance? And, how is it possible that Keisha, who by no means meets Sydney's definition of perfection, leads a very happy and fulfilling life? The same approach can be applied to the patient with concerns about balding (i.e., why is it that we know many bald men who are happy?). The answers to these questions help us see that, while not meeting the social performance and appearance standards we set for ourselves can be disappointing, it doesn't have to be a recipe for fear. It becomes a recipe for fear and a life with repeated false alarms when people (erroneously) believe that failing to realize these desired outcomes has catastrophic consequences.

Recognizing that we as clinicians are prone to making erroneous appraisals just like our patients facilitates accurate assessment and helps ensure that we remain focused on the goals that the patient and clinician set for treatment. That is, Sydney wants to feel less lonely, which may require she gives up on some of her perfectionistic tendencies.

6.2. Intervention Targets

Caring less about the evaluation of others, or being genuine in social situations, is a behavioral outcome that reflects a shift from seeing others' evaluations as harmful to viewing these evaluations as lacking true danger. We would argue that attending to this behavioral outcome provides better clinical guidance and ultimately better clinical outcome than attending to any symptom-based assessment instrument tapping social anxiety symptom severity (see Chapter 9). That is to say, reductions on a measure like the Liebowitz Social Anxiety Scale (LSAS) or scoring below the cut-off for recovery (i.e., 30) certainly provide an indication that a patient is achieving his or her treatment goal (i.e., he or she experiences less fear and reports less avoidance across a number of performance and social interaction situations). However, we can be more confident that we have knocked out social anxiety and related disorders when a patient treats and enters most of these situations with more of a laissez faire attitude. Indeed, he or she can afford to because *most* social situations are relatively meaningless as they have very little impact on our functioning and that of others. We find the following exercise helpful to illustrate this principle to the patient and to begin the conversation about setting intervention targets.

Clinician: We have been talking about your goals for treatment, and it is clear to me that we will be successful when you are able to expand your social activities and when you experience less fear when you are the center of attention. Before we move on to discussing the approach we will take to achieving these goals, can you quickly list the best five social interactions for the past year?

Sydney: Uhm, top five, let me see. Wait, that's hard. What do you mean?

Clinician: Just tell me about five interactions that you remember, as in they were important.

Sydney: Okay. Hmmm. I am thinking maybe my birthday dinner with my sister. That was fun. I am not sure that it was important though. I mean I have had several of these dinners with her, and they are all reasonably important to our relationship. Maybe the annual budget meeting at work. I had to present on how we as a firm were doing regarding the retention of junior staff. Now that I think about it though, we ended up not having to use that information for the annual report, so I guess it wasn't that important after all. I think you are going to have to give me some more time to come up with the top five. Maybe I can tell you when I see you next week.

Clinician: Great. I really like doing this exercise. Your reaction and responses are not so different from what I typically get from others. Do you have any idea why I am asking?

Sydney: A memory test, showing that I am not that smart?

Clinician: Not really. I love hearing your answer because it simply illustrates that most—and I mean almost all—social interactions you and all of us engage in are relatively meaningless. At the end of the year, we may remember a handful, and typically only when prompted or reminded, and the others are long gone from our memories. This fact tells us something important. That is, if almost all social interactions are meaningless, then it makes sense to start treating most situations as such. That's a departure from the approach that you take. You are telling me that you spend days anticipating a meeting and hours following a meeting to rehash what was said and done. This approach makes sense if the meeting carried some significance. But, you're telling me that almost all don't. What do you think?

Sydney: I get it. It seems silly to devote so much energy every time if in the end it doesn't matter. I recognize that I am overdoing it. Gosh, I can only imagine what it would be like if I dealt with social situations the way I deal with, let's say, what to choose for dinner. The problem is, though, that I really do feel like it matters when I am thinking about the situation or when I am in it. Sometimes I think, I do not need to spend another hour of this, but then my heart is racing, and I have this feeling in my gut that motivates me to do it anyway. Not sure how to change that.

Clinician: That's why you are here. I want you to identify someone you know who is the Michael Jordan of social situations, that is, someone you know for whom being in social situations is effortless. Can you think of someone?

Sydney: Oh yes. Keisha, my sister. I hate, sorry for saying that, seeing her at parties. I am the one standing by the door, while she is right in the middle of the room talking to strangers and really doesn't care. And it's not like she is all that attractive or so poised. I mean look at me. She just is not intimidated by anyone.

Clinician: What do you think about the fact that Keisha just treats these situations like they don't mean anything?

Sydney: I don't know. I have always been jealous of her for being able to go about these situations with so much ease. I just think that I'll never do that. I have too much to lose.

Clinician: I know that it feels like that. What you are stating is at the center of social anxiety are your concerns about your appearance and performance. You recognize, on the one hand, that it shouldn't matter, but you have a strong feeling, on the other hand, that tells you it does. I am going to propose that Keisha has few concerns and is not experiencing anxiety in social situations because she acts in a way that sends a message to the brain that she's safe. Without preparation or hesitation, she dives in, trusting that she will come out fine. I am not saying this to point the finger. Instead, I am highlighting the power of action, which should get us excited. That is, when you will go about

> social situations differently, not just once, but repeatedly and consistently, you will start seeing them as not that important and thus knock out your fear. Let's talk about how you can get there.

It's unreasonable to expect that a patient like Sydney will take this exercise to heart and then do a 180 on her action plan and processing as it relates to performance and social interaction situations. As she states, her habits are strong and are mostly guided by her feelings rather than her rational thinking. At this point in treatment, we can only ask for Sydney to be open-minded to the idea that relinquishing control (i.e., giving up on safety behaviors), trusting that harm is unlikely, is what it takes to overcome an anxiety problem. Our task as clinicians is to develop a set of exercises that motivates her to move toward that end.

6.2.1. Consider Intervening on the Likelihood Bias First

We conceptualize the recurrence of false alarms as a product of likelihood and cost biases. The likelihood bias reflects the overprediction of the occurrence of a negative outcome, whereas the cost bias refers to the overprediction of harm should the negative outcome occur. When people are the feared cue, likelihood bias typically takes on the form of excessive concerns about being perceived or judged as incompetent or inadequate (e.g., showing visible symptoms of anxiety, poor performance). The cost bias is evident when a patient appraises such outcomes—being perceived or judged as incompetent or inadequate—as having disastrous consequences (e.g., living in isolation, failure in life).

As we have discussed in Chapter 3, the default approach to knocking out false alarms is to go right to targeting the core fear. When a patient fears living in isolation because he or she believes preventing that requires always giving people a positive impression, he or she needs to learn that poor performance can indeed lead to negative judgment, but that such negative judgment, despite being undesired and unpleasant, does not have critical implications. Establishing unconditional safety or removing the "what ifs" for this patient ultimately involves being playful with performance. That means, letting go of preparation, winging it more, and making mistakes on purpose. Albert Ellis's story about how he overcame his fear of rejection by asking over 100 women out and being rejected by most is a nice example of what are called "social mishap" exposures. So, why not start there? We cannot argue against starting there. In fact, we recommend beginning the conversation about targets discussing the default.

> So, we have talked about what it takes for you to finish treatment knowing that you got it out of your system. That is, when you start seeing your interactions

with people much like you see, let's say, eating lunch—as in I do this every day and it is not that important—you are in the position to make your social and work life much more rewarding. Imagine for a minute that you truly cared less like Keisha does; can you see that you're more likely to attain your goals—or get what you want—at work and in your social and romantic life.

Let me tell you the story about Albert Ellis, one of the founders of cognitive behavioral therapy. He was terrified of rejection. To get over this, he decided to go to the Bronx Botanical Garden every day for a month and when he saw a woman sitting alone on a bench he approached her by sitting next to her and starting a conversation. He relinquished control by telling himself that he was okay with the worst outcome—the feeling of being rejected. Apparently, about a third of the women he approached simply got up and left. The remainder stayed and talked with him. He ended up only with a few dates (and some that didn't show), but, most important, he was able to see that what was so difficult for him to do didn't have any catastrophic consequences (e.g., no one attacked him, called the cops, or made a scene). At the end of the one-month experience, Albert said that he was no longer afraid of rejection. On top of that, he felt like he had some good practice and felt like he was more effective in communicating with women.

I love telling this story for a few reasons. First, it shows the power of what we call mishap exposures. That is, putting yourself in the situation that leads to negative judgment and, when doing that over and over again, seeing that it's relatively meaningless. Second, what most of us desire—making good impressions—is much easier to accomplish when we get rid of the fear of rejection. When we no longer care so much about that, we can be more genuine and that facilitates performance. So, I think you get what I'm saying. I'd say, let's not worry about performance now, but trust that will come once we treat the fear of rejection.

Also discussed in Chapter 3, our patients vary greatly with respect to willingness to engage in demanding exposure exercises. Some patients will respond to this prescription telling you to bring it on. Others, though, may recognize the value of mishap exposures, but eagerly decline. They will tell you they are not ready for that and are unwilling to try. It's when this occurs, that we recommend clinicians target the likelihood bias first.

6.2.1.1. Trap 2: Inadvertently Strengthening the Cost Bias

Again, there is incredible value in having a sense of mastery. That is, we all like doing things we are good at and appreciate it when we see that the effort we put into learning new things pays off in enhanced performance. A patient like Sydney often would like nothing less than coming away from therapy feeling better about her skills and how she appears to others. Certainly, there may be merit in highlighting to Sydney the discrepancy between her imagined and her actual performance/appearance (see Figure 6.1). Doing so will reduce the likelihood bias—"I don't appear as anxious as I thought." Here also lies the trap of reinforcing the cost bias. Specifically, by focusing on disconfirming concerns about being rejected, we may inadvertently communicate to the patient that performance is indeed crucial and rejection must be avoided at all cost. One way to avoid that trap is to name it and frame the initial exposure practice as a method to help the patient become more flexible in terms of his or her thinking rather than to simply illustrate that performing well is more likely than he or she thought (and that that is important). Applied to Sydney, the following script may be useful in this regard.

> I understand that being playful with rejection feels like it is too much for you now. You're not alone in that. Many patients I work with will say that they can work up to mishap exposure practice that but they prefer to start slowly. When that's the case, we find that there can be merit in working on what we call the *likelihood bias* first. The likelihood bias reflects the tendency to overestimate anticipated negative outcomes in social situations. For you, it is the concern that when you enter social situations, that you will appear anxious. I know that this is an overestimation on your end, and we can do some work together for you to also recognize that.
>
> You can see, though, that I am a little concerned about heading in that direction. That is, if we start focusing on performance, we run the risk that you will start valuing it more as opposed to less. So, the challenge for us will be to help you stay on course—moving toward caring less. We can ensure that when we are careful about processing the exercises. Don't get me wrong, it will be great for you to come to see that some of things you're imagining are way off, but it will be even better when you use these exercises to learn that you've simply been off when it comes to making predictions about harm in general. When I say this, I hope you don't take it as criticism, but instead as a message of hope. That is, we can be very successful together as it just takes getting you to think more accurately in these social and performance situations.

6.3. Exposure Practice

6.3.1. Basic Conditions

Regardless of the target of the intervention—likelihood or cost bias—exposure practice will be most effective for Sydney when it meets the following conditions:

(1) *Systematic.* The careful planning of exposure exercises involves input from Sydney about selecting intervention targets and how to best develop the exercises to engage these targets (see Section 6.2).
(2) *Deliberate.* Practice will be in Sydney's control, as in she determines the time and circumstances of exposure practice, allowing her to have agency in her improvement.
(3) *Prolonged.* The duration of the practice or ending the exposure exercise is determined by achieving a goal instead of the drive to escape, as this allows Sydney to relate differently to false alarms.
(4) *Repeated.* It is primarily when Sydney repeats exercises within and between sessions that will she learn that safety is unambiguous and unconditional.

I know that you understand the goals of exposure therapy and how it works as we discussed this in the last two sessions (see Chapter 3). Let's talk a little bit more about what this actually means for how we put it together in our sessions.

As you can tell, our work is going to be very collaborative. I want you to think about this as a course where you and I develop goals or targets—like we just did—and then design the exercises that help us achieve these goals. That way, you are going to be very active in leading the effort to help you get rid of your fears. As I watch for progress, I'll be excited when you start coming to the sessions with ideas of how we can tweak an exercise to best serve your needs.

The exposure practice will be different from the efforts that you have been putting in every week. That is, I know that you are great about enduring various social interaction situations, but these often just happen to you randomly as opposed to you seeking them out on purpose for practice—or with the intent to learn, as will be the case in our sessions. In addition to being deliberate, exposure practice will be prolonged. What I mean by that is that we want to make sure that the exposure to the situation you fear is long enough in duration such that you can practice responding differently to the fear. As in, rather than escaping or avoiding the situation when it gets uncomfortable, you want to get practice doing nothing—or "relaxing with the symptoms"—and thus allowing fear to dissipate. The last key principle of effective exposure therapy is repetition. We don't want to do an exercise just once trusting that is sufficient to develop this new safety memory. Building new memory takes practice! That's why we will make sure that you repeat the exercise several times during as well as in between sessions. This is where homework comes in. The mission is for you to get bored with it. Once you're bored with it, we can be sure that you no longer see the situation as dangerous.

6.3.2. Personalizing Practice

Exposure practice always involves a simulation. The aim is to develop an exercise that approximates a real-life situation that can activate the patient's core fear, thus providing an opportunity to develop a safety memory by:

(1) practicing responding to the fear differently (i.e., not doing anything about it), and
(2) gathering discomfirmatory evidence (i.e., attending to information that violates the patient's harm expectancies).

We determine the specific parameters of the practice (e.g., type of activity, patient's actions, clinician's actions, context) based on the target for intervention (which is always guided by the case formulation). Hence, while it's relatively easy to select an activity to activate the fear (e.g., develop a hierarchy of feared situations/cues), it takes some careful planning to personalize the practice to ensure that it yields good and productive learning.

6.3.2.1. Trap 3: Missing the "What Ifs"

Let's consider a patient we treated for spider phobia to illustrate the importance of personalizing exposure practice. Singh was a 28-year-old male who presented for treatment because he found himself running to the closet to get his gun to kill a spider he had spotted in his bed. Even though he didn't pull the trigger, he recognized his reaction was excessive, and his wife urged him to get help. During the assessment, it became clear that Singh feared all spiders regardless of size or color but was particularly wary of the ones that make sudden movements. The unpredictability bothered him because he felt like he would not have time to protect himself should he be attacked. On top of that, he was bothered by the fear sensations, worried that he might do something he would regret if he had a panic attack (e.g., get into a fight, break furniture).

Singh's hierarchy of feared situations was pretty straightforward. Lower on the hierarchy-ranked imagining was seeing pictures or watching movies of spiders. In the middle of the hierarchy were activities like going to a pet store and seeing live spiders, whereas on the top of the hierarchy was holding a spider.

We started the intervention with prolonged and repeated presentation to spider pictures and movies. Singh's Subjective Units of Distress Scale (SUDs) level was a steady 60 and did not move with repeated practice within the session. This may seem surprising because for most patients with spider phobia, such exposure practice leads to boredom pretty quickly. So, why didn't that happen for Singh? It turned out that the fear of fear was getting in the way. That is, Singh indicated that even when he experienced a lower-level fear response, like a SUDs of 25, he worried about it escalating to a panic attack, which then would result in some regrettable behavior. What Singh was telling us is that his sense of safety around pictures and movies of spiders was conditional (i.e., I feel safe but *what if* I have a panic attack?).

If we don't attend to the "what ifs," we risk engaging in unproductive exposure exercises or, even worse, moving away from exposure therapy altogether because of the false conclusion that the patient is nonresponsive.

Singh's experiences with exposure practice were not surprising given the fear-of-fear sensations operated prominently in the case formulation. It guided us to alter some of the exposure parameters. Specifically, it was clear that Singh needed repeated experiences with panic attacks in the context of spider stimuli to learn that safety in the presence of spider-related stimuli was unconditional. To that end, Singh agreed to:

(1) make the practice of undetermined length (*duration*),
(2) lean into the feelings rather than to fight them (e.g., stating aloud "Bring it on"; *patient's actions*), and
(3) allow the clinician to play loud sounds at different times to stimulate panic (interoceptive *context*)

When we personalized exposure practice by varying these parameters, Singh was able to practice relating to panic differently and thereby learned to see that the harm he associated with spiders was very unlikely.

6.3.3. The Parameters

As we make clear in the example of Singh, effective exposure practice requires that we have to tweak the exercises to engage the target. As we prepare to work with someone like Sydney, who needs to learn that being the center of attention is safe, it is helpful to consider the key parameters for exposure to people and how they can be varied to yield an optimal learning experience for her.

6.3.3.1. Activities

Activating the fear of people requires that our patients enter the situations where they are the center of attention and subject to criticism. Generally, the following types of activities are suitable for either in-session practice or otherwise homework practice (which has fewer restrictions).

- Presentations (e.g., reading aloud, giving a report, public speaking)
- Interactions (e.g., talking to strangers, introductions, initiating a conversation, asking someone on a date)

- Being observed (e.g., eating/drinking/telephoning in public, writing/reading while being observed)
- Inconveniencing others (e.g., asking for directions, disagreeing, turning someone down, talking to people in authority)

In addition to using the LSAS, which lists 24 common activities patients with fear of people commonly fear and avoid, it can be helpful to ask your patient to develop a hierarchy of feared situations. Individualizing the activities, or specifying conditions under which the activities produce fear, will likely help you and the patient be more efficient with subsequent practice. Again, the case formulation (see Figure 6.1) offers a starting point for identifying meaningful cues/activities.

> From your responses on our assessment [i.e., we use the LSAS in our clinic; see Chapter 9], I can get a sense of situations that provoke fear. I can see that speaking up at a meeting is hard as is telephoning in public. I would like for you to spend some time adding to this list and make one that is more specific to you. As you can see, the LSAS lacks specifics about the situations. I know that returning goods to a store, for example, may provoke different levels of fear depending on the nature of the store, the item that is returned, etc. So, what I would like you to do over the next week is come up with a list of specific activities—think specific places, specific people, your anxiety state, etc.—and rate each of them on SUDs (0–100) and desire to avoid (0–100).

6.3.3.2. Patient's Actions

In general, the patient's actions during exposure practice should be centered on embracing the fear. This is a deviation from his or her habit, which is to fight the fear and find ways to avoid it or escape from it. Embracing the fear during exposure practice includes:

- attending to the feelings and sensations (e.g., stop distraction, lean into the feelings, name the feelings),
- relinquishing control (e.g., remove safety behaviors, let clinician or partner/friend direct practice, include surprises), and
- opposite actions (e.g., make postural modifications to signal safety, intentional mishaps).

Our experience is that clinicians often overlook the importance of patient's actions or ignore them altogether. Arguably, the positive effects of exposure therapy depend in large part on how the patient responds to his or her fear reaction. A patient who learns to lean in and a clinician who can facilitate that will be most likely to be successful.

When discussing patient's actions during exposure practice, we start by describing the ideal scenario, recognizing again that a patient may choose to adopt a gradual approach.

> Remember that your behavior and actions are key in the fear cycle. Getting you back into the situations that you fear is important but crucial to seeing *fear reduction* is what you do when you experience the fear. Consider, for example, the differences in responding to fear in three patients undergoing exposure therapy for flying phobia. The first patient gets to the airport four hours in advance, drinks three beers, stays on the phone with a friend to distract himself before take-off and keeps his eyes closed, gripping the seat for the entire duration of the flight. The second patient gets to the airport with sufficient time to make it through security, recognizes his fear response is a false alarm, treating it like he treats a back pain ("There it is, my heart is pounding, a classic sign of the false alarm") and focuses on acting normal even though he doesn't feel normal when in his seat. That means he recognizes the symptoms, yet engages in conversation, reads a book, watches a movie, etc. The third patient does everything that the second patient does, but in addition, he attends to his posture—he makes sure that it's similar to what it is when he sits at home watching TV—and he is playful with the fear, like he is telling himself to bring it on and he is wishing for turbulence. You can see that, depending on what the patient *does* during exposure practice, the experience can be sensitizing like it is for Patient 1, or it can be therapeutic like it is for Patient 2, or highly therapeutic like it is for Patient 3. Let's spend some time identifying the key actions we want to attend to when you engage in exposure practice.

Sydney's responses on the SAFE provide nice direction in terms of developing targets for her behavioral responses during exposure practice (see Figure 6.1). Specifically, we would encourage Sydney to fade preparation (e.g., excessive grooming, checking, and rehearsing), lean into the fear, and act in a way like she does with, let's say, her sister (even though she feels uncomfortable and she can't). It is important to recognize that the responses on the SAFE assume that the patient has good insight and is aware of subtle avoidance maneuvers. Our experience is that the first exposure exercise serves as a behavioral test, allowing us the verify responses on the SAFE and identify additional avoidance maneuvers and opposite actions to be targeted during subsequent practice.

6.3.3.3. Clinician's Actions

As clinicians, we serve multiple roles. First, we are a major source of support for our patients. Patients open up to us and tell us about their vulnerabilities, and we provide a setting where this is safe. Second, we serve as coaches, guiding our patients through demanding learning experiences with the aim to develop new safety memories. Changing habits is difficult. Patients come to us because they know they need to change their habits, but they need someone to help them do it. These roles can be complementary, but they can also pose challenges and, if not handled correctly, may undermine the effects of exposure therapy. Facilitating optimal learning during exposure therapy requires that clinicians are aware of and act on the following dos and don'ts.

Dos

- Encourage (e.g., give pep talks, show unyielding optimism, model the action, problem-solve).
- Acknowledge (e.g., validate emotions, show empathy, point out how efforts will pay off).
- Highlight (e.g., make the patient aware of discrepancies between anticipated and actual outcomes, provide feedback, point out progress within and across sessions).
- Reward (e.g., offer praise, develop a reward structure to reinforce homework practice).
- Process (e.g., review the aims of practice, review what happened, review what was learned, discuss the implications of new learning).

Don'ts

- Escape (e.g., supporting stopping practice before achieving the goals, expressing concerns about fear being too taxing).
- Reassure (e.g., responding to repeated requests to assure the patient that nothing bad will happen [i.e., becoming a safety signal], exhibiting concern/anxiety while observing practice).
- Delay (e.g., postponing exposure practice thus reinforcing a patient's avoidance tendencies, hesitant to push the envelope on exposure exercises).
- Rely (e.g., trusting homework noncompliance will resolve itself without intervention).

6.3.3.4. Context

Recognizing the patient's tendencies to process exposure practice contemplating the "what ifs" (i.e., "I know this is easier now, but I am not sure whether I would feel that way if you were not here"), we as clinicians have to prioritize varying contexts in exposure practice. That is, if we repeat exercises across different contexts, we are more likely to help the patient build memories of *unconditional* safety. Relevant contexts for patients like Sydney who fear people because of the perceived consequences of being rejected include but are not limited to the following domains.

External Contexts

- Clinician/clinic (e.g., clinician, office setting, time of day, day of the week).
- Work/school (e.g., number of people, "rank" of people [perceived importance], type of gathering [formal or informal]).
- Relationships (e.g., closeness [perceived importance], setting [formal or informal], type of activity).

Internal Contexts

- Stress (e.g., perceived demands in major life domains [e.g., relationships, work, finances, health]).
- Fatigue (e.g., feeling tired, bodily symptoms of fatigue, cognitive impairments associated with fatigue).
- Fear activation (e.g., SUDs, type of bodily sensations and their intensity).
- Visible symptoms of anxiety (e.g., blushing, sweating, mind going blank).

We recommend taking a few minutes during the session to educate the patient on the importance of varying contexts during exposure practice and to start working with him or her to identify key contextual factors and ways to manipulate exposure practice to systematically include these variables. Again, the goal is to engage in unambiguous safety learning, defined as safety learning that includes the contextual factors that would otherwise signal danger. In Sydney's case, it's important to validate social anxiety symptoms as true alarms after instances of discrimination, racism, and micro-aggressions. Doing so guides effective exposure practice (i.e., only targeting false alarms), as well as possible problem-solving (i.e., how to cope with true alarms).

Using the memory node model from previous chapters, Figure 6.2 depicts learning the safety of public speaking that does and does not include the event of facial blushing. In the left frame, facial flushing is left out of the safety learning and still signals fear if it occurs during public speaking. By including induced blushing (see following discussion) in exposure exercises, the clinician can help ensure that safety is learned that includes this cue.

> We've been talking a great deal about ways to undermine the effects of exposure therapy. I keep hammering on the importance of the "what ifs"—the tendency of most patients to question whether what they have seen or learned during practice will actually generalize to the situations that really matter. Obviously, our goal is for you to feel safe when you're the center of attention regardless of

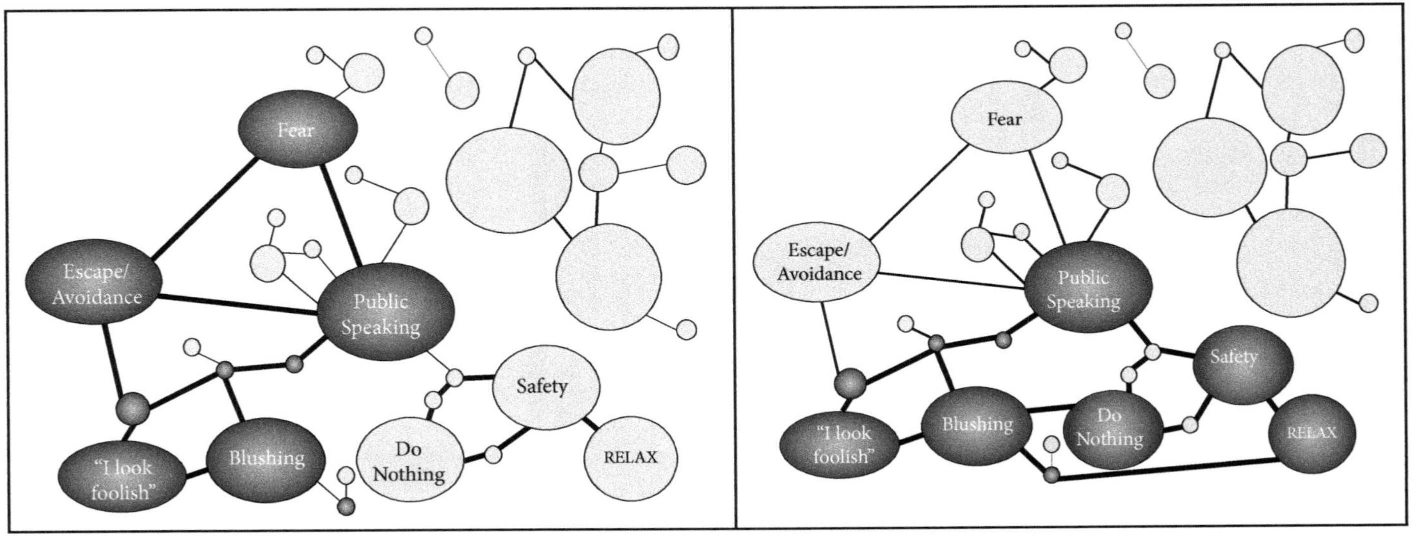

Figure 6.2 Left panel illustrates the continued linking of blushing with threat, with little learned safety in this context. Right panel illustrates more unambiguous learning of safety, incorporating blushing into the learned safety memory node.

Table 6.1 Assessing and Varying Context for Sydney

Domain	Applicable	Contextual parameter	Manipulations
External			
Clinic/Clinician	√	Clinician present	When Clinician is not present
	√	Therapy room	Outside of the office
		Time of day	
	√	Day of the week	On Fridays after a long week
Work/School	√	No. of people	In small groups
	√	Rank of people	With senior partner present
		Setting	
Relationships		No. of people	
	√	Rank of people	When around males with high perceived social status
	√	Type of gathering	While on a first date
Internal			
Stress	√	Work	During busy times at work
		Relationship	
		Finances	
		Health	
Fatigue	√	Feeling tired	After staying up at night
		Bodily symptoms	
		Cognitive impairments	
Fear Activation	√	SUDs	When SUDs are >90
	√	Symptoms	After caffeine administration to induce feeling jittery
Visible Symptoms of Anxiety	√	Mind going blank	After niacin administration to induce blushing
		Sweating	
		Blushing	

Note. SUDs = Subjective Units of Distress Scale.

> the setting, the type of people, or the way you feel. To get there, we need to make sure that we vary what we call contextual factors—the nature of the situation, how you feel—during the practice. Let's take a look at this form [see Table 6.1] and complete this together.

As you can see in Table 6.1, considering the various contextual parameters in tandem with the case formulation leads to some clear strategies (e.g., manipulations of internal and external cues) that can be employed to help ensure that the effects of exposure practice generalize.

6.3.4. Progression

Exposure therapy is goal oriented. You attend to two major markers or "yardsticks" for success as you decide how to progress or sequence exercises.

(1) The first marker is the degree to which the patient is learning safety. Once a patient becomes bored with an exercise and can articulate that his or her feared outcome is unlikely, it's time to move on to different cues.
(2) The second marker, which is often more relevant at the beginning of treatment, is the degree to which a patient sees that exposure can be used effectively to highlight maladaptive habits (i.e., safety behaviors, cognitive inflexibility, misappraisals) and, importantly, engages these treatment targets to promote fear extinction. Instead of violating harm expectancies, success in this domain is violating (negative) treatment expectancies; that is, the patient can articulate the goals of exposure therapy and, importantly, believes that approaching fear and changing his or her response to it is critical to getting rid of false alarms.

6.3.4.1. First Exercise

For Sydney, who is reluctant to engage in exposure therapy, even though she understands the model, demonstrating that she is no different from others (i.e., she also will experience the positive effects of exposure practice) is a key first goal. A first exercise for Sydney can involve having a conversation (see Box 6.1). Sydney has difficulty initiating conversations, especially if it involves males. Rather than selecting a neutral topic, asking Sydney to talk about herself and a topic that increases a sense of vulnerability (discussing her dating history) is more likely to generate the symptoms that she often experiences in social interaction situations. For the exposure practice to be successful, it will be important not only for Sydney to see that persistence or staying in the conversation will

Box 6.1 Sydney's First Exercise

Patient: *Sydney* **Date:** *7-6-2018*

Target threat appraisals (use response on ***the ASC***):
Feared outcome: *showing visible symptoms of anxiety* Rating: *80%*
Feared outcome: Rating:
Feared outcome: Rating:
Feared outcome: Rating:

Goals
Experiencing moderate fear (SUDs level of 50), "relaxing" with fear symptoms, attend to disconfirmatory evidence

Situation/Cue
❑ Social interaction: Bodily sensation:
❑ Social performance: Other cue(s): *Someone of the opposite sex*

Manipulations to Achieve Match to Fear Cues
❑ Interaction/performance topic: *Brief conversation about dating*
❑ Duration (specify minutes):*undetermined*
❑ Fade other safety cues/behavior (s) (use response on the SAFE): *Avoiding eye contact*
List targeted safety cue/behaviors:
❑ Induction of interoceptive sensations (list):
❑ Social errors/mishaps (specify):
❑ Feedback: videotape feedback

Set specific and achievable behavioral goal (based on goals and manipulations above):
Introduce yourself to a stranger (male) and engage him in a conversation about dating and your experience. Attend to fear symptoms and lean in. Do not stop the conversation because you want to escape the fear.

Note. ASC = Appraisal of Social Concerns scale.

allow for the symptoms to run their course but also will provide some clear evidence that her predictions are off the mark. To facilitate meeting the latter goal, we can use Sydney's phone to video record the exposure conversation, focusing on the specific aspects of her appearance she is most concerned about (e.g., blushing, sweating, speech rate, etc.). Complementing the exercise with video feedback, which highlights the discrepancy between her imagined appearance/performance and actual appearance/performance, has the potential to disconfirm the specific threat appraisals and more generally highlight her tendency to make errors in her predictions.

Steps

(1) Establish and agree on goals and determine the specifics of the activity (see Box 6.1).
(2) Initiate the exercise attending to the following:
  a. *Repetition.* Repetition here simply means to start over from the beginning repeatedly. The patient does not have to vary the content. In fact, the instruction can be to repeat the conversation in a similar fashion, using the same sentences, thus sending the signal that the exercise is not about performing well but instead about learning that when responding differently to symptoms, fear will dissipate.
  b. *Patient's actions.* Encouraging the patient to lean into fear attending to his or her (subtle) actions that point to a tendency to avoid or escape. As you notice the patient is fighting the fear, you may stop the exercise briefly, highlight the actions (and posture) that are getting in the way, practice "acting" normal (i.e., "What would I see on a video recording if you were feeling comfortable") and then instruct the patient to start again from the beginning engaging in the appropriate or therapeutic actions.
  c. *Patient's SUDs.* Ask the patient about SUDs prior to starting the exercise and then again periodically during the exercise. Use SUDs as a marker for ending the practice (e.g., as the signal that the person has learned to feel more safe, to ensure that the patient is not ending the practice to escape the feelings of fear).
  d. *Patient's thoughts.* As you attend to SUDs levels and their change, you may ask the patient about his or her thoughts. Relating his or her thoughts to SUDs (and their change) highlights the premise of exposure therapy; that is, the patient will be feeling more comfortable as he or she learns to appraise the cues as safe. Identifying the thoughts that fuel his or her fear also aids in modifying the exercise if needed (i.e., "What do you need to see for you to believe that you don't appear as anxious as you think?").
(3) Feedback and processing. As mentioned previously, the "risk" of providing videotape feedback to Sydney is that it can inadvertently reinforce her belief that a good performance has to be achieved at all times. Therefore, setting up the goals of videotape feedback are critical. Specifically, you may reiterate that the principal aim of videotape feedback (for ease, using a

smartphone video function) is to illustrate that she tends to make errors when she predicts the outcomes of social interaction and performance situations. You want to ask Sydney to first tell you what she imagines seeing on the recording before playing it. Here, it's importance to ask about specifics (i.e., how can we tell you are blushing, what about the speech rate was problematic and when did that occur and how long did it last, etc.). Then, when viewing the recording, make sure that Sydney focuses on what the video recording displays instead of what she felt during the practice. This instruction orients the patient to attending to new information as opposed to possibly reinforcing a negative feeling. After viewing the recording, engage Sydney in a discussion about the evidence for and against her predictions. Finally, ask Sydney the following two questions:

a. What did you take away from the exercise?
b. How was the exercise useful; that is, how does it help you as you will encounter these and related cues in real life?

(4) Homework assignment. Enlist Sydney's help in designing an assignment that reinforces and helps generalize the learning that occurred during the session. An initial homework exercise for Sydney would be to repeat the conversation with her brother.

6.3.4.2. Later Exercises

Once Sydney is on board and has experienced some initial successes, exposure practice can move toward targeting the cost bias and also incorporate addressing her body image concerns. Exposure practice targeting the cost bias involves being playful with mistakes. Guided by the case formulation (see Figure 6.1) and the context assessment (see Table 6.1), Sydney would benefit from exposure exercises such as the following:

- Giving repeated brief speeches in front of coworkers without wearing make-up and after taking niacin (200 mg). Because niacin induces facial flushing, this exercise facilitates learning that, even though uncomfortable, appearing uncomfortable and anxious does not have catastrophic consequences.
- Going on a date and discussing her least favorite physical features after having only slept a few hours the night prior. Highlighting (instead of hiding) the perceived flaws in her physical appearance sends a powerful message to the brain that being judged on these features is not important. Doing this while also feeling fatigued adds to the benefits of this exercise,

because Sydney will learn that she can effectively manage fear regardless of fatigue.

An important addition to the previously described steps is that processing of exposure practice targeting the cost bias requires a specific plan to address negative postevent rumination that is typical in patients with rejection sensitivity. Especially after "underperforming," or in this case making mistakes on purpose, Sydney likely will recount the experience repeatedly, emphasizing the negative feelings and her perceived evidence of failure and rejection. As such, postevent rumination can get in the way of cementing new learning of safety and therefore needs to be anticipated and remedied.

One of the things you've told me is that you, like many other people who fear rejection, tend to replay interactions in the hours and sometimes even days following an event. We have talked about how this gets in the way of overcoming an anxiety problem. You find yourself focusing on how bad you felt and confirming that you made so many mistakes. This gets in the way of you fully experiencing that, regardless of how you perform in most social situations, you will be fine. So, our goal is to remove this type of rumination and, instead, help you learn to shift your focus from being in the past to being more in the here and now. I anticipate that you are going need the most help in this area following exposure practice that involves making mistakes on purpose. So, I want you to be prepared and talk about how we can go about intervening on this.

Preparation is the first step. This treatment is all about relating differently to your habits. One way to do that as it relates to rumination is to anticipate that it will happen such that when it begins you can welcome it with a smile. "As in, there I go, this is what I do, my habit is to relive a negative experience and beat myself with a stick." Recognizing it and naming it will help you relate to the process differently and gives you an opening to make a choice: Do I delve in further, or do I shift and move on? Moving away may be made easier by reading a series of questions that you have handy in the notes app on your phone. Questions like, "Did I ever benefit from spending more time on recounting the event?" "Just because it feels like the right thing to do, what do I know about letting my emotions drive my actions?" "Have there been times that I regretted it when I didn't spend time reliving the experience?" These questions help underscore the futility of rumination and promote a willingness to change the habit. The key to being successful in moving away at that time is shifting your environment. It's unlikely that you are successful resisting the pull when you stay in the same position. So, if you're lying in bed or on the sofa, get up and walk around. If you're sitting at your desk staring at a screen, pick up the phone and call your sister. Shifting your environment comes with a new set of cues that draw your attention. It forces you to step away from rumination and provides an opportunity to let go, trusting that doing so is, indeed, in your best interest.

Now, like with everything we do here in treatment, repetition is critical. We cannot expect that you will be effective resisting the inclination to ruminate at all times. So, this will be something that you will practice, and you and I will identify barriers and discuss strategies for overcoming these during our sessions.

6.4. When to Do What

Personalized exposure therapy implies that the selection and sequencing of activities and the speed and progression of treatment vary across patients. In our view, the clinician who achieves the best outcomes with exposure therapy is one who is flexible and makes decisions on what to do and when to do it based on the case formulation and the patient's responses to session activities (e.g., assessment, education, exposure practice). That said, we recognize that it is helpful to provide clinicians with a general roadmap including a prototypical session (see Table 6.2) and prototypical intervention (see Table 6.3).

Table 6.2 Prototypical Session

Task	Activities	Time
1. Agenda setting	• Discuss session goals • Determine session activities	5 min.
2. Assessment	• Review symptom severity • Review what has been learned	5 min.
3. Review of homework	• Review experience • Review outcomes relative to goals • Trouble-shoot barriers	5 min.
4. Practice	• Education • Exposure practices • Cognitive strategies	30 min.
5. Review and homework assignment	• Review what has been learned • Discuss how learning can be applied • Determine homework	5–10 min.

Table 6.3 Prototypical Intervention

Session	Aims	Activities
1	• Develop initial case formulation	• Assessment
2–3	• Refine case formulation • Socialize patient to exposure therapy	• Assessment • Education
4–6	• Socialize patient to exposure practice • Experience initial success with exposure practice	• Develop initial exercise • Practice initial exercise
7–11	• Building the safety memory	• Exposure practice
12	• Termination	• Review progress

6.4.1. Prototypical Session

Clinicians enter each session with a specific goal that can be stated in the form of "If today's session is successful, I want the patient to leave having learned that . . ." Barring emergencies that require crisis management and thus a different format (e.g., support, assessment, and plan for immediate action), all treatment sessions will be structured such that the purported goal can be achieved. The session starts by setting an agenda, orienting the patient and clinician to the session goals and how to attain them. We check in with the patient, review his or her week and progress both in terms of symptom improvement as well as retention of learning.

> Each week, I am curious what the effect was of the last session. I am pleased to see that you continue to report improvement in your symptoms [see LSAS scores] and how you think about situations before you enter them [see ASC scores]. Tell me again what you took away from our last exposure practice and, importantly, how it affected you this week?

Next, we briefly review the homework. We reinforce homework completion by offering praise ("Awesome, job. I know it's hard to fit in). When the patient did not complete homework, we spend some time troubleshooting ("What got in the way?" "What can we do differently this week to ensure you will get it done?" "Do we need to make the homework easier in any way?") and make sure we implement new strategies for subsequent homework assignments.

The bulk of the session will be devoted to the next step in helping the patient learn safety in response to his or her fear cues. Early sessions focus on getting the patient ready for exposure practice. Activities include assessment to refine the case formulation, education to socialize the patient to exposure practice, and discussion of parameters to develop specific exposure exercises. The teaching in subsequent sessions centers on the acquisition of fear extinction or the building of safety memories. It involves the delivery of clinician-guided exposure practice. Practice is always followed by a review bringing it back to the larger agenda.

> Today, we set out to have you leave the session seeing that exposure practice can work. We developed an exercise and you completed it. I'd like to know from you how you feel like we did in terms of achieving the session goals. What did you learn and, importantly, how do you think that will affect you when you wake up tomorrow.

Finally, the session ends with a homework prescription that aims to promote the cementing of the safety memory. Hence, the emphasis is on rehearsal and application. In earlier sessions, homework includes a review of education (see Chapter 10), where we may ask patients to teach their friends, family, and/or significant others. Following sessions that involve exposure practice, homework always involves some sort of repetition of what has been practiced in the session. The aim is to repeat and remove the what ifs by varying contexts.

6.4.2. Prototypical Intervention

Table 6.3 depicts a prototypical session-by-session treatment plan for a patient like Sydney. Personalized exposure therapy begins by working together with the patient to (a) understand why the patient experiences fear, (b) to make clear how exposure practice can be used to overcome fear, and (c) how to best fine-tune practice to the specific needs of the patient (sessions 1–6). Once the patient has some evidence that exposure therapy doesn't just sound good on paper but actually can work for him or her, he or she is ready to push the envelope on exposure practice working toward building memories of unconditional safety (sessions 7–11). Termination involves a review of progress and a plan to continue to tackle false alarms in the same fashion, should they (re) emerge.

Table 6.4 Troubleshooting

Problem	Reasons	Strategy
No shows	• Poor socialization to exposure therapy	• Education, initial successful exposure practice
Homework nonadherence	• Poor socialization to exposure therapy • Busy schedule • Avoidant due to anxiety	• Education, initial successful exposure practice • Schedule specific times • Break exposure homework into smaller component steps, after additional in session rehearsal
Failure to identify safety behaviors	• Seeing false alarms as true alarms	• Consult with colleagues to validate case formulation
Lack of symptom improvement	• Reinforcing instead of violating harm expectancies • Failing to teach unconditional safety	• Education, processing of exposure practice • Ensuring basic conditions are met, varying exposure practice parameters

6.5. Troubleshooting

Throughout this book and the chapter, we have described the dos and don'ts as they relate to exposure practice and pointed to common traps and how to avert them. Table 6.4 summarizes these as it relates specifically to the fear of people.

6.6. Conclusions

In this chapter, we have applied the approach to preparing, implementing, and processing exposure therapy to the fear of people. We have described the general patterns and habits seen in patients who present with rejection sensitivity but emphasized the importance of considering the factors that are unique to the case and how they inform treatment planning and delivery. The aim was to make clear and illustrate that the case formulation, which includes the processes that maintain false alarms as well as the patient's thoughts and approach to therapy, drives (a) what we target in the intervention and (b) what we go back to for decisions on how to fine-tune exposure practice and how to progress through treatment. Chapters 2 to 4 provide complementary information on initial assessment, case formulation, and tracking of progress throughout treatment.

7

Fear of Thoughts, Images, and Trauma Memories

7.1. Overview

In Chapter 5, we emphasized how difficult it is for people to fear their own emotional experience/bodily sensations. The fear is of what lies within. Individuals with this fear feel the ongoing vulnerability of awaiting activation of that fear by the next relevant situation. This description is also apt for fears of thoughts, images, and memories. Again, the fear lies within, and it is often activated by relevant outside cues.

Consider the case of posttraumatic stress disorder (PTSD). Understanding the fear of one's own memories is a central for understanding PTSD. The trauma was horrific, and that horror established the trauma memory as something to fear in its own right, in part because the experience of rekindled fear can be so overwhelming. The memory of the trauma and the storm of emotions it brings engenders a host of avoidance strategies: Trying not to think about the trauma, trying to avoid external reminders of the trauma, and trying not to experience emotions associated with the trauma. Moreover, when internal or external trauma cues are encountered, the trauma memory is activated not as a historical threat, but as a *current* threat. The perceived current threat may be defined by fears of being overwhelmed by the emotional storm, fears that the trauma may somehow reoccur, and/or fears of losing control more generally (see the Posttraumatic Cognitions Inventory measure described in Chapter 9 that can be used to assess the patient's perceived threats following trauma). Figure 7.1 provides a memory node perspective of the link between the trauma memory and a current danger interpretation.

Given what has been covered thus far in this book, it's clear that the clinician has a wide range of exposure targets for treating the fear of trauma memories that is central in PTSD. There are external cues that lead to the trauma memory, there are internal emotional cues that lead to the trauma memory, and, reasonably, there are imaginal cues of the trauma—all of these cues have the potential to activate the trauma memory and thus can be targeted for treatment. For any of these exposure targets, the task is the same: Provide a patient with opportunities to develop a sense of safety with this trauma memory, so that it no longer evokes a

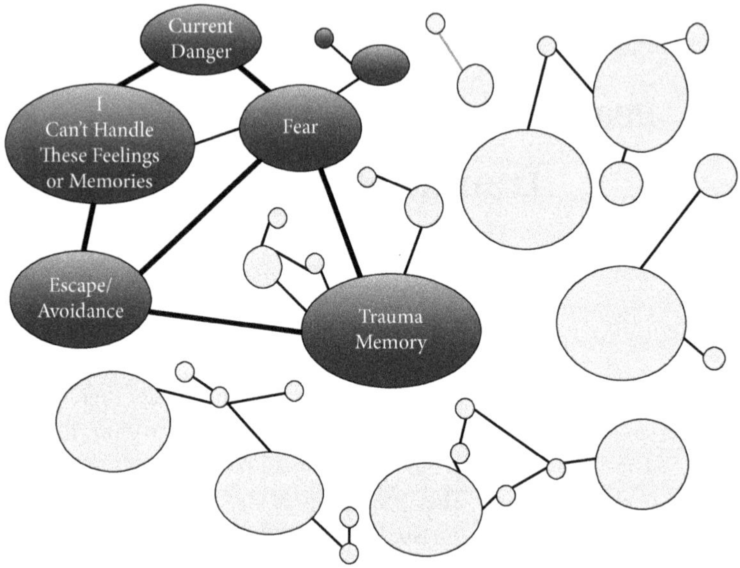

Figure 7.1 Memory node model of current danger interpretations to the trauma memory.

current danger interpretation. What replaces the current danger interpretation? We find that patients often describe a sense of calm sadness that replaces the very active anxiety, avoidance, and coping attempts that are part of PTSD. The trauma happened, but with treatment it became an event in the past to be mourned. And the memory of this past event is no longer regularly evoked by everyday cues. Figure 7.2 shows this resolution of the trauma into an appropriately historical memory instead of a harbinger of current threat.

We find that the idea of thinking about PTSD as a phobia of the trauma *memory* aids clinicians, as it guides them to design exposure practice to engender a shift from perceiving the *memory* as dangerous to appraising the *memory* and resulting emotions as both safe and tolerable. In the same way, clinicians can benefit in their treatment planning and implementation from considering the possibility that thoughts and images, much like memories, can cue phobic reactions because patients falsely link these internal experiences to danger. That is, the undesirable thoughts (e.g., thoughts of dying alone or one's children dying, thoughts of failure, thoughts of harming others) or images (e.g., blasphemous images, uncomfortable sexual images, images of hurting others or oneself) that are central in generalized anxiety disorder (GAD), obsessive-compulsive disorder (OCD) and related disorders (e.g., social anxiety disorder,

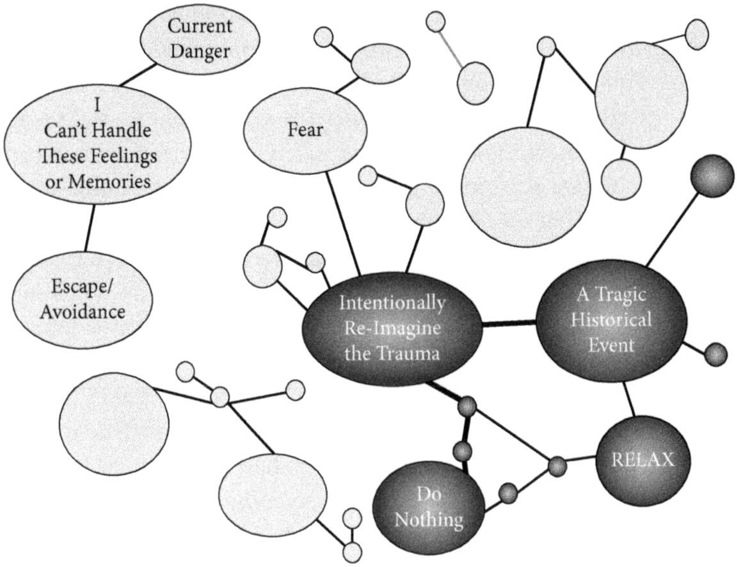

Figure 7.2 Memory node model showing reduced activation and alternative meanings to the trauma.

illness anxiety disorder, body image disorder, etc.) can become overwhelming, recurrent, and difficult to dismiss when one attaches a sense of threat to these thoughts or images. Our task as clinicians is to help patients knock out these false alarms, providing them with opportunities to learn that, while one's own cognitive content (e.g., thoughts, images, and memories) can be painful, unusual, or unwanted, it is not harmful.

7.1.1. Factors That Enhance the Fears of One's Own Cognitive Content

There are several pathways to enhanced fears of one's own cognitive content. We mention three individual difference variables or traits here that function as amplifiers and become a target of intervention when intervening on fears of thoughts, images, and memories. Assessment strategies for these factors are discussed in Chapter 9.

(1) *Anxiety sensitivity*. Recall that in Chapter 5 we reviewed the role of interoceptive exposure in treating PTSD precisely because fears of emotional

cues are frequently part of the broader fears within PTSD. Indeed, for patients with elevated anxiety sensitivity, certain moods (e.g., anger, depressed mood, panic) and (related) somatic arousal (e.g., increased heart rate, sweating, dizziness) can enhance the salience of expected/imagined scenarios or memories. Establishing safety memories for these patients requires that we also reduce their fear of emotions and bodily sensations (see Chapter 5 for specific strategies).

(2) *Intolerance of uncertainty.* The unwillingness to tolerate the *possibility* that negative events may occur in the future leads to overattention and to attempts to manage every risk. For those with elevated intolerance of uncertainty, it is not the *probable* risks, but the *potential* risks that are attended to, often in the form of a "what if" thought. That is, the intolerance of uncertainty (a cognitive trait leading people to attend to and seek safety signals for possible dangers rather than just the probable dangers) is a transdiagnostic risk factor for worry, obsessions, and avoidance, as well as a host of maladaptive attempts to neutralize threat. The intolerance of uncertainty helps transform thoughts and worries about harm into false alarms. The result is that the person is motivated to neutralize this perceived threat (false alarm), setting the stage for overvigilance, worry, obsessions, compulsions, avoidance, and other safety behaviors. Relating differently to predictions of risk is a core focus of treatment when the aim is to reduce fears of thoughts, images, and memories.

(3) *Thought–action fusion.* An additional risk factor for establishing the overimportance and dangerousness of thoughts and images is thought–action fusion. Thought–action fusion refers to the belief that having unwanted thoughts or images must increase the likelihood of the perceived dangerous outcome to occur (e.g., "Because I have thoughts of harming my parents, I will end up harming my parents"; termed *likelihood thought–action fusion*) or is just as bad as experiencing the perceived outcome (e.g., "Having sexual images of God means that I am a bad person"; termed *moral thought–action fusion*). Because thoughts are assumed to portend behavioral action, the thoughts themselves become dangerous and become the target for strategies to neutralize threat (e.g., attempts to block thoughts, neutralize thoughts with counter-thoughts, or avoid situations or other cues that evoke thoughts or reparative actions to make up for thoughts). A fundamental aim of exposure therapy when targeting the fear of thoughts and images is to uncouple this cue–threat appraisal relation. Indeed, exposure is successful when patients are curious about rather than afraid of their own cognitive content (see Chapter 4).

7.2. The Role of Imaginal Exposure in Treating Fears of Cognitive Content

For fears of trauma memories or thoughts/images of negative outcomes, one of the central learning tasks is to establish a sense of safety with one's own cognitive content. At times, this involves clarifying the striking difference between thoughts, memories, and images of an event and the actual occurrence of event in the world (e.g., differentiating memories of an assault vs. an actual assault, thoughts of the death of a loved one vs. actual risk of death, and thoughts of being fired vs. the actual risk of being fired). Imaginal exposure provides a perfect fit for this task for at least three reasons:

(1) The exposure occurs in the same modality as the fear cue: An internally generated event (e.g., an imagined scene, the memory of the trauma) is used as exposure for a feared internally generated event (e.g., a thought, image, or memory).
(2) Imaginal exposure allows for therapeutic exposure that would not be possible with in vivo strategies. Whereas the memory of a trauma is a false alarm, actual trauma is a true alarm. What do we do with cues that accurately identify true harm? We escape and engage in problem-solving to make our world more safe. True alarms are a reason for protective action. Yet, *thoughts, memories,* and *images* of these and other true alarms are valid targets for exposure. Indeed, they are simply false alarm reflections of the true alarm, and they can be readily generated by imaginal exposure.
(3) The act of purposefully generating and holding a traumatic image or feared thought or image in mind is a directly opposite action to the avoidance behavior associated with many of these fears—for example, the avoidance of trauma-related thoughts or feelings of PTSD (Criterion C), or strategies to neutralize thoughts or images (e.g., compulsions to repeatedly say "Hail Mary's" to neutralize a blasphemous thought in OCD). In this way, imaginal exposure for fears of cognitive content is directly comparable to in vivo exposure for situational avoidance (e.g., going to a mall for a patient with agoraphobic avoidance): It directly helps patients to undo avoidance responses that define the disorder. Indeed, imaginal exposure involves confronting the imagined scenarios (e.g., thoughts and images) or evoked images of the feared cues. The thoughts, images, and trauma memories produce false alarms, and thus exposure can be applied to teach safety in the presence of thoughts, images, or trauma memories as well as tolerance of the evoked emotions.

7.2.1. Planning for Imaginal Exposure

The first step to implement imaginal exposure is to conduct a careful evaluation and the development of an initial case formulation (see Chapter 3). As always with anxiety and its disorders, we want to answer the question "Of what is the patient afraid?" This question should be prominent in the clinician's mind during the intake and initial sessions. In addition to utilizing the questionnaires that tap common threat appraisals related to thoughts, images, and trauma memories (see Chapter 9), the following questions are helpful in the case formulation and development of targets for exposure:

(1) *What cues start the process* of frightening thoughts, emotions, bodily sensations, and maladaptive responses (avoidance or neutralizing behaviors)? Cues can be internal (memory, thought, image, bodily sensation) or external (trauma reminders, situations, people).
(2) *What frightening thoughts follow* the presentation of the cue? What is the core threat (e.g., "The memory will make me go crazy"; "I will die of cancer"; "My child will be killed")?
(3) *What emotions and bodily sensations does the patient have* in response to these cues (e.g., fear, heart racing)?
(4) *What does the patient do* (safety behaviors) when he or she has these thoughts, emotions, and bodily sensations (e.g. avoidance, drinking, rituals, reassurance seeking)?
(5) *What are the results* of these responses? What are the short-term effects (e.g., reduced anxiety)? What are the long-term effects (e.g., reduced quality of life)?

The downward arrow technique can be a useful strategy in determining the core threat that fuels the fears. For example, consider Malik, a 53-year-old businessman who reports his fears intensify when he has to fly. You can start by asking him, "What are you afraid will happen?" Malik replies, "I'll be away from my spouse," which prompts you to ask, "What is so concerning about that?"

As illustrated in Figure 7.3, you arrive at a legitimate core threat when you can discuss that the perceived outcome is one that would be threatening to most people. How do you decide whether you have arrived at a legitimate core threat? Consider the "10 judges" metaphor. Imagine we lined up 10 judges selected at random from the community. We present each perceived threat in the downward arrow figure until all 10 judges are convinced that the outcome would be truly frightening. If you stopped at a fear of flying, perhaps one or two judges would agree. Likewise, not all judges may feel frightened if their spouse left them. Some of them may not have a spouse. Some may already wish they were

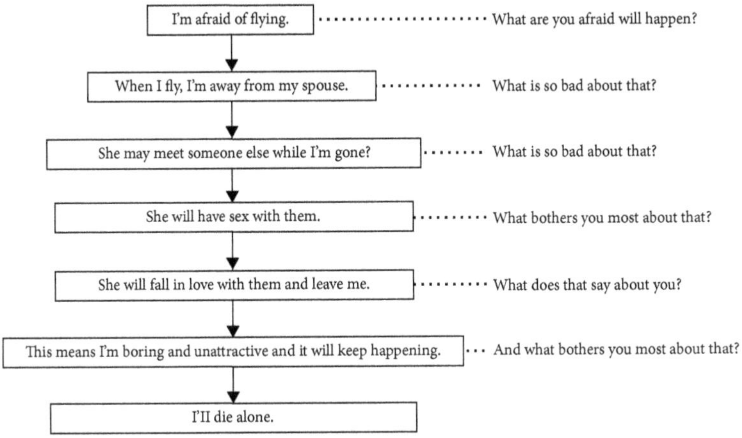

Figure 7.3 The downward arrow technique.

divorced. And some may think they would be fine and bounce back, eventually finding someone else. But all 10 judges are likely to fear dying alone with no one in the world who cared about them. The script developed to guide the imaginal exposure requires that we know the patient's core threat. Indeed, only a script guiding imaginal exposure that centers around the core threat (as opposed to more "surface" level concerns) will result in the safety learning that helps your patient knock out his or her fears.

7.2.2. Developing a Script for Imaginal Exposure

For fears of trauma memories, imaginal exposure involves recounting the trauma memory (detailed in the following discussion). For fears of thoughts and images, imaginal exposure requires drafting a script that can guide imagery. The script should be drafted like a movie that is as realistic as possible. The goal is to have the patient view the memory, image, or thought as a real event without maladaptive avoidance strategies but with efforts to differentiate the memory, image, or thought from an event. Said differently, the goal is to have the imaginal image be a good match to the thought, image, or memory that the patient is avoiding. This cannot be accomplished without input from both the clinician and the patient. The patient is obviously the expert concerning his or her core threat. The clinician, however, assumes the important role of coach by helping the patient attend to the details that allow for imaginal exposure practice that can optimize safety learning. Consider the following introduction to imaginal exposure for Malik, the patient with GAD who experiences heightened anxiety when traveling.

I would like to introduce imaginal exposure today—why we do it and how we do it. We use imaginal exposure to confront catastrophic outcomes you fear that we cannot access in real life. For example, you mentioned that due to your traveling, your spouse may meet other people, leave you, no one else will love you, and you will die alone. You are afraid of the idea of dying alone. Obviously, you also know that that unwanted outcome is a product of your imagination; that is, you feel like it is likely to happen at the time you're traveling but you recognize that your feelings and thoughts are often not accurate. To get you to relate to this negative outcome differently, much like you can with all kinds of other possible negative outcomes, I will ask you to imagine the series of events that lead to this worst-case imagined feared outcome. Now, I am not going to ask you to just do this once and just at random like you may have done before. I know that can be sensitizing. Instead, I will ask you imagine this scenario systematically, deliberately, for a prolonged period of time, and repeatedly. When you do it that way, you will learn to get bored with this scenario and, as a result, develop a renewed sense of safety around all kinds of cues related to the thought of dying alone.

To generate the movie, we will first create a script for the scenario. Once we're happy with the script, we will audio record it so that you can have it available for repeated practice.

An effective imaginal exposure script includes:

(1) cues (e.g., thoughts; situations; bodily feelings including sights, sounds, smells, tastes, and sensations; and emotions);
(2) threat appraisals;
(3) images;
(4) feelings (e.g., emotions, sensations);
(5) behaviors used to neutralize the perceived threat (e.g., safety behaviors, covert/overt rituals, compensatory behaviors); and
(6) ultimate confrontation with the internally generated threat.

Using a computer or tablet, the clinician may start writing the script, modeling the process of generating an effective narrative of the feared event for the patient, and then ask the patient for his input.

Clinician: Let me get us started. I'm sitting in the airplane flying to London. The air is warm and smells stale. I feel that my stomach is warm and unsettled because I know Amy will be going out with her friend Stacy and will probably meet guys who are more attractive and interesting than me. I am ordering another drink to help with my nerves. As I drink, I decide to email Amy in the hopes she will tell me she is at home. I repeatedly check my email over the next hour. She must be out already. Now, help me continue the story. Pick up where I left off.

Malik: I'm not sure I'll do this right but OK. Here goes. I'm now in my hotel room in London. I should be enjoying the room, but I have a sinking feeling something is wrong. Just then the phone rings. I answer but hear no voice. Then in a quiet trembling voice, Amy says she has been sleeping with someone for over a year and she is filing for divorce. Even though I feared this coming for years, I feel adrenalin rush through my body. I feel like my life is over. After returning home to the empty house, I decide to start a new life. I go out with my friends, but it's not like it was in college. No women talk with me. They look disgusted when I try to strike up a conversation. My friends become tired of me always asking them for reassurance and drinking heavily whenever we go out. I start just staying home—hopeless. I grow old staying in the same house and lose my job as I stopped being able to sell myself in meetings and in sales. The house is so empty. I hear nothing. It is dark in here and cold. I'm in a bed in a room with no TV and on hospice. There is no one there. I never had children, and each night I go to sleep and don't know if I'll wake up. I feel like the air is thick and hard to breathe. I'm sure I'm close to death. I wish someone were here with me or cared about me. I slip into death alone and afraid.

The next step is to record the script for Malik to listen to in session and for homework, using his smart phone or some other mobile recording device. Some research suggests recordings in the patient's rather than the clinician's voice may be more effective in terms of generating the imagery, but this is something to discuss with each patient. Either way, it is important that the pace of the recorded content is slow enough so a patient can follow along easily. Thus, make sure that whoever records the script incudes pauses between sentences to help increase the drama and realism and to allow time to fully imagine the scene.

7.2.3. Delivering Imaginal Exposure

Much like exposure to other cues described in the previous chapters, the key to effective imaginal exposure practice is that you activate the fear memory and help ensure that your patient does nothing to try to neutralize the fear, thus allowing for an unambiguous safety memory to develop ("I can have this image and be okay with it; I don't have to manage the image or how it can make me feel"). To facilitate engagement and activation of an effective image, you may instruct your patient to sit back and close his or her eyes, allowing him or her to picture the scenes as vividly as possible. Before playing back the recoding, you can ask for a Subjective Units of Distress Scale (SUDs) rating (i.e., "What is your SUDs now?"), which you will repeat again after the recording ends (i.e., "What was the highest level of SUDs you experienced during practice?"). We recommend repeating this exposure process for at least 30 minutes each session.

The processing of the new safety learning at the end of exposure can be initiated with the question, "What was that like for you?" Coaching can then center on comparing the patient's actual experience to what he or she expected, drawing attention to what was learned. The session is successful when the patient draws the conclusion that distressing thoughts, images, and memories are just that—thoughts, images, and memories. They are not the same as real life in the present moment. The homework prescription involves repeated practice with the same recording, making sure that the patient varies important contextual parameters (e.g. home vs. away from home, morning vs. at night, when rested vs. when tired), aiming to establish a new safety memory that is unconditional.

7.2.4. Progressing with Imaginal Exposure

The decision to stick with the same exposure script, to adjust the script, or to develop a new script is based on how the patient responds to the imaginal exposure practice. We consider the following parameters:

(1) *In-session behaviors.* As we have emphasized in previous chapters, a patient who learns to do nothing in response to a false alarm is on his or her way to develop a new safety memory. Hence, we recommend that patients achieve this outcome (e.g., remove safety behaviors, adopt a posture signaling safety) before altering the cue (e.g., modifying the script, developing a new script).

(2) *SUDs activation.* An increase in fear during practice (relative to before) indicates ongoing appraisal of threat and thus suggests that the script can still be useful for exposure practice. Once the patient no longer "reacts" to the script, he or she is bored with it, indicating that his or her fear has extinguished.

(3) *SUDs decline.* Especially early on in the intervention, it can be helpful for a patient to see the clear benefits of the courage to confront the feared cue(s). Highlighting SUDs decline within a practice session (i.e., decline in peak SUDs across multiple trials) and across practice sessions (decline in peak SUDs across practice days) can increase motivation to engage in future practice.

In as much as the initial script serves to initiate new safety learning, it also helps you and the patient fine-tune the case formulation and thus guides you in how to move forward. Variations in SUDs during the script may simply validate the core fear themes (e.g., if Malik reports he almost panics when he hears "I wish someone were here with me or cared about me") or can point to other possible fear themes that have not been previously identified (e.g., if Malik reports high SUDs around imagining women not responding to him when he strikes up a conversation, it may be that his fears are also fueled by rejection sensitivity [see Chapter 6]). Scripts that are the focus of subsequent practice involve either modifications to the original script that emphasize and elaborate on scenes that produce the greatest fear activation or new scripts that target other fear themes. In addition, clinicians may want to focus on certain phrases that have overlearned negative meaning (e.g., "I will be abandoned"). Targeted exposure (i.e., having the patient repeat this one phrase 60 times for each of three exposures) can be helpful in sapping the meaning of the phrase and in reducing the degree of threat in the overall script developed by the patient.

In summary, imaginal exposure emerges as a particularly fitting strategy for treatment of fears of thoughts, images, and memories. It uses evoked images to help the patient develop a sense of safety with the thoughts, images, and memories. It has advantages over in vivo exposure because it is specific to the false alarm rather than any true alarms—allowing for exposure when in vivo exposure may not be appropriate or feasible (e.g., for combat traumas, contracting a disease, dying alone, harming someone). Nonetheless, in targeting the fears of one's own cognitive content, there is often a role for situational exposure (see Chapters 3 and 6) for peripheral cues: Those cues that do not predict danger but are nonetheless fused with the feared outcomes. Likewise, there may be a role for interoceptive exposure to separately target emotions as noted in Chapter 5. We discuss this combination strategy next.

7.2.5. Complementing Imaginal Exposure with Interoceptive and In Vivo Exposure

Intrusive thoughts and memories are, of course, cued by a wide range of situational (e.g., seeing a church for blasphemous thoughts or images, seeing a hospital for thoughts of dying, or seeing a kitchen knife for concerns about harming others) as well as internal (e.g., feelings of anxiety, guilt, and/or sadness) events. Accordingly, the relevance and/or intensity of imaginal exposure practice can be supplemented by use of additional cue exposure as a prelude or context for imaginal exposure (e.g., an object or smell related to the fear). Also, in vivo and interoceptive exposure can be used to extend safety learning for other types of cues feared in patients who present with fears of thoughts, images, or trauma memories. To clarify, two core strategies for combining imaginal exposure practice with exposure to external (in vivo) or interoceptive cues are concurrent use and sequential use.

(1) *Concurrent use*. Certain external or internal contexts intensify fears of one's own cognitive content, and thus clinicians may want to conduct imaginal exposure under these more "salient" conditions. The "what if" question (i.e., I feel safe, but what if . . .") introduced earlier in the book can guide you to develop a list of relevant contexts for your patient. Consider, for example, the possibility that Malik would develop a stronger safety memory if he conducted imaginal exposure practice immediately after he watches a brief YouTube video of checking into an empty hotel room. Similarly, the patient who developed PTSD following rape will learn to feel more safe around the memory after she has conducted imaginal exposure practice while standing near the park where the rape happened, smelling the cologne of the assailant, and experiencing racing heart.
(2) *Sequential use*. Imaginal exposure may be followed by in vivo exposure practice tasked specifically to eliminate vestigial avoidance behaviors, once fears of one's own cognitive content has been reduced. A listing of avoided activities, perhaps organized hierarchically (from least avoided/lowest SUDs rating to most avoided/highest SUDs rating) can help you and the patient decide on selecting relevant activities for in vivo exposure practice. In the same way, a patient may be able to engage more fully in imaginal exposure focused on the trauma narrative following interoceptive exposure practice that has helped reduce fears of intense emotions and related somatic arousal (as detailed in Chapter 5).

7.2.6. Prototypical Session and Intervention

The flow of each exposure session (Table 7.1) and intervention (Table 7.2) for targeting fears of thoughts, images, and memories is similar to that we discussed for other cues (see Chapters 3, 5, and 6). Each session begins with setting an agenda and session goals (e.g., socialization, building/strengthening safety memory). The case formulation and initial experiences with exposure practice will help you decide on what exposure exercise to practice in the session. We recommend reserving much of the session for practice, recognizing that,

Table 7.1 Prototypical Session Content for Targeting Fears of One's Own Cognitive Content

Task	Activities	Time
1. Agenda setting	• Discuss session goals • Determine session activities	2 min.
2. Assessment	• Review symptom severity • Review what has been learned from the last session	3 min.
3. Review of homework	• Review homework exposure practice • Decide on exposure practice for current session	5 min.
4. Prepare for exposure practice	• Develop exposure exercise • Varying external and internal context if necessary	10 min.
4. Exposure practice	• Listening to recording • Practicing doing nothing in response to fear • Repeat	25 min.
5. Session review and homework assignment	• Review what has been learned • Discuss how learning can be applied • Discuss homework	5 min.

Table 7.2 Phases of Treatment as Applied to Fears of One's Own Cognitive Content

Phase of Treatment	Aims	Activities
1	• Develop and refine case formulation • Socialize patient to exposure • Experience initial success with imaginal exposure practice	• Assessment • Education • Rehearsal of nonresponse to imaginal exposure • Possible "pretreatment" with interoceptive exposure
2	• Learning to "do nothing to manage symptoms" when exposed to feared cues the context of additional relevant contexts (e.g., external and internal contexts)	• Diversify exposure practices
3	• Learning that safety is unconditional	• Safety behavior fading • Conduct relevant imaginal and in vivo exposure

especially in the beginning, effective exposure practice (e.g., ensuring adequate fear activation and therapeutic responding to fear activation) requires coaching. That coaching extends to the processing after each practice that facilitates the cementing of new safety learning.

Phase 1 centers on developing a personalized treatment plan and socialization (see Chapter 3). Although personalized exposure implies that the sequencing and protocol length varies across patients, we recommend beginning with imaginal exposure, but stress that effective safety learning may require concurrent exposure to external cues or bodily sensations (Phase 2). Alternatively, the core fears the patient presents with may require that you complete in vivo or interoceptive exposure practice either before or after you begin imaginal exposure (see Section 7.2.5.). Phase 3 focuses on strengthening the safety memory attending to varying contexts, the targeting of vestigial avoidance behaviors and making room for value-guided activities.

7.3. Transdiagnostic Considerations

Now that we have laid out the general principles of planning for and implementing exposure therapy for fears of one's own cognitive content, we can turn to a discussion of specific additional strategies unique to each of the three cognitive cues when they become a target of intervention. For ease, we decided to provide case examples for GAD, OCD, and PTSD to discuss the treatments of fears of thoughts, images, and memories, respectively. We would like to re-emphasize, however, that targeting these feared cues is not limited to these three anxiety disorders. For example, in the clinic we treated Eric, a 48-year-old male nurse anesthetist, who presented with insomnia disorder. Despite having had a successful career involving multiple long (i.e., 36+ hours) shifts, Eric had developed a fear of the thought of making a lethal mistake at work. This thought and associated images had resulted in "fatigue sensitivity," which along with a number of safety behaviors (e.g., sleeping mask, ear plugs, calming tea) caused him difficulty falling asleep. It wasn't until Eric felt safe around *intrusive thoughts and images* of making mistakes (did not emotionally react to false alarms) at work that his sleep was restored. Similar processes, where thoughts, images, or memories cue fears, are evident in other anxiety (e.g., specific phobia, social anxiety disorder) and related (e.g., illness anxiety disorder, body dysmorphic disorder, anorexia, bulimia nervosa, sexual dysfunctions) disorders.

7.4. Treating Fears of Thoughts in GAD

Let's return to Malik, the 53-year-old married businessman coming to the clinic for help with his GAD. Now, although it may be clear to the treating clinician that he has a "thought phobia," Malik does not have that insight when he presents. Consider his description of the anxiety he experiences:

> I've been an anxious guy my entire life. I'd say my anxiety is always about a 6 out of 10. I know I worry more than others when something is going on like being in a meeting at work or going on vacation. I just feel keyed up and on edge even when nothing is happening. That is, I really worry about so many things, like whether I will be a in a car crash, who will take care of my children after I die, or whether other people worry like this. And then, I start worrying about my performance at work and losing my job and so on. My best description of my anxiety is that it feels like when you're alone at night walking to your car in a dangerous part of town and you'd like to get to your car quickly. I feel like this all the time. I feel like my nervous system is just turned up and wish there were a way to turn it down. I can feel my anxiety in my stomach and my shoulders. As a teenager and college student, I drank a lot. I remember the first time I had three beers and thought, this must be how normal people feel. Of course, drinking three beers all the time wasn't a good or even possible strategy. I still drink though if I can. I've tried relaxation, counseling, exercise, and medications, and none of them seem to work, although my wife says the medication has helped some. My other therapists asked me what I worried about but I worry about everything. It's a moving target. I'm not sure what else you could do for me but I figured I'd give it a try.

Scoring a 15 on the Generalized Anxiety Disorder 7-Item Scale (GAD-7; see Chapter 9), Malik's symptom severity is characteristic of patients with GAD as is his presentation. Indeed, he describes experiencing the classic for GAD "worry chains"—a series of worries that follow one after the next by switching topics (see Figure 7.4)—and also recognizes that that he has difficulty tolerating uncertainty (his score on the Intolerance of Uncertainty Scale is 47; see Chapter 9).

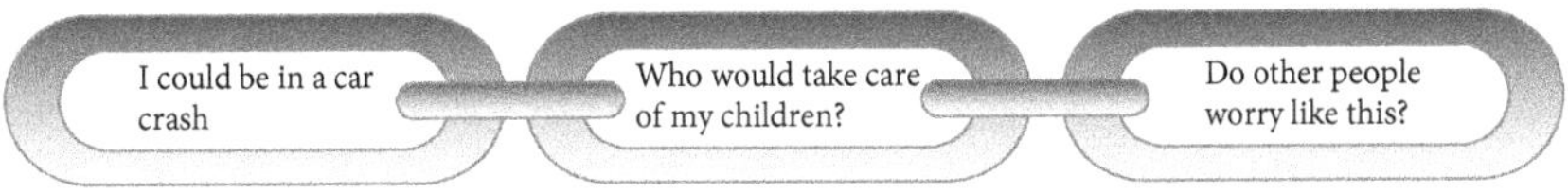

Figure 7.4 Worry chain.

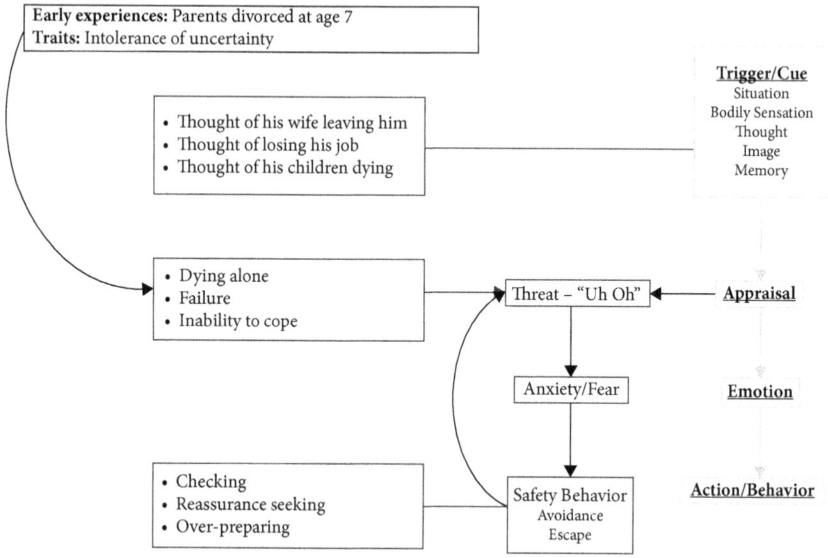

Figure 7.5 Malik's case formulation.

Interestingly, although he thinks he worries about "everything," a review with his clinician reveals three themes of harm that link the cues/thoughts and his safety behaviors (see Figure 7.5):

(1) *Cue*: The thought of his wife leaving him
Perceived threat: Dying alone
Safety behaviors: Calling his wife, checking her location on his phone, asking her for reassurance, watching her behavior when in public for indications she is interested in others

(2) *Cue*: The thought of losing his job
Perceived threat: Failure
Safety behaviors: Going to work early and staying late, avoiding meetings with his boss, saying yes to all requests, excessive list-making

(3) *Cue*: The thought of his children dying
Perceived threat: Inability to cope with the loss of his children
Safety behaviors: Calling his children daily, watching their locations on his phone, sending them news stories about violent crimes in their cities

You can see that what are benign cues (i.e., thoughts of undesirable outcomes) are particularly triggering for Malik because he views these as initial signals of the inevitable dangers he believes he will face later in life (e.g., failing, unable to cope, and ultimately dying alone; see Figure 7.5). His safety behaviors, while giving him the immediate sense that he is managing his perceived danger, maintain the danger interpretation. As is true for many patients with GAD, Malik's worry "style" (see Figure 7.5) serves the same function as his other safety behaviors. Specifically, this mental coping strategy often gives him the sense that he is engaging in problem-solving yet, because it stays at the surface, bouncing from one thought to the next, never resolves his core fears but instead continues to fuel them. Malik's intolerance of uncertainty amplifies the emotions he experiences when events do not go as expected (e.g., a meeting starts late, his children do not pick up the phone, his wife cancels a dinner date) and promotes his tendency to exert control when possible, thus maintaining the vicious cycle.

7.4.1. Targets for Intervention

An adaptive safety memory for Malik is not about him being okay with being unable to cope, failing, or dying alone. These are negative outcomes that yield true alarms we all should aim to avert. Instead, treatment for Malik is about providing him with a sense of safety around *thoughts* of these undesirable outcomes and to the ability to tolerate uncertainty around these feared themes much like he does around other themes. It's important to note that the clinical evaluation with Malik reveals that he describes his marriage as a loving relationship and he has been able to move up the ladder at work receiving continuous praise. Hence, what differentiates Malik from others is not his true risk in these life areas, but the way in which he reacts emotionally and behaviorally to his worries about these life areas.

7.4.2. Developing an Intervention Plan

Patients with GAD, like Malik, go from one worry to the next in rapid succession and tend to feel "on guard" at all times. Even daily hassles can serve as cues for anxiety and avoidance. Important life tasks are neglected as a result. The chaotic environment that results seems to confirm that the world is dangerous, which, in turn, reinforces the drive to remain hypervigilant. Breaking the cycle seems insurmountable to them and potentially dangerous. This ambivalence to give up worry is an early target in therapy. To address this, psychoeducation on the cost–benefit analysis of worry and avoidance behaviors can be helpful, as detailed in the following discussion. Once the patient agrees that his or her worry strategy is maladaptive (i.e., you have successfully oriented him or her to the exposure therapy model), you have formed the basis to start breaking the cycle with imaginal, in vivo (and possibly interoceptive) exposure, sticking with one fear theme at a time. Processing focuses on a cost–benefit analysis of living life and engaging in value-guided actions, which are inconsistent with the actions that have been driven by the worries and underlying fear themes (i.e., avoidance). Thus, we recommend that exposure therapy for fear of thoughts that are seen in GAD includes the following two additional specific strategies:

(1) education about worry as a maladaptive coping strategy, and
(2) cost–benefit analysis of alternative strategies.

7.4.3. Education about Worry as a Coping Strategy

As discussed earlier, worry serves a coping function for many patients with GAD and fears of thoughts. Engaging in worry can give these patients the sense that they are problem-solving, staying alert, and making sure that they avert negative outcomes. Although they recognize that worrying is ineffective particularly in the long-term (i.e., they have never truly felt that they are "on top of it"), it's difficult to consider moving away from worry activity (i.e., "I know it doesn't help, but it feels right to do it"). It's helpful if you can highlight this habit and help a patient see that shifting attention away from worry will be an important strategy along with the fading of other safety behaviors to overcome the fear of thoughts. For example, the clinician may say:

> I recognize the value of worry. For example, I can tell you when I receive an email that my grant was not funded, I immediately turn my attention to my personal and lab financial states and find myself quickly considering the worst-case scenarios. This can then turn into worrying about my staff and family and lead to me wanting to go online checking my bank account and reaching out to others about possible ways to obtain funding. This type of worry activity, even though it's taxing, gives me the sense that I am problem-solving. I know, though, and I realize the next day that the time spent thinking about these things and seeking reassurance doesn't deliver. In fact, I've learned, through practice, that actively disengaging from this activity—that is, forcing myself to do something else than worrying when I receive bad news—works better for me. That is, it gives me back valuable time and has shown me that most of these

what appear to be true alarms are actually false alarms and deserve to be treated as such.

I have found that it's helpful to think about worry as a habit that, because it feels right, is difficult to give up. Learning to recognize the force that pulls you in to engage and, importantly, to be effective in disengaging is a major goal of our work together.

The tactics to teach disengagement from worry are similar to those targeting postevent processing that we discussed in Chapter 6 and include training (a) awareness of the maladaptive habit (e.g., recognizing it, naming it), (b) preparedness to question the habit (e.g., developing the dialogue to consider resisting the habit), and (c) readiness to implement actions that facilitate disengagement (e.g., shifting the environment, listing of productive behaviors).

7.4.4. Cost–Benefit Analysis of New Behaviors Alternative Strategies

In line with the message that worry is a maladaptive coping habit is the emphasis on developing behaviors that compete with worry and have the potential to be rewarding. Giving up any safety behavior is challenging as it forces patients to take a leap of faith, trusting that anticipated feared scenarios will not play out. Spending less time on worry (the "misguided" attempts to problem-solve) becomes more appealing when a patient can point to gains he or she has made in terms of engaging in activities that he or she finds enjoyable and/or important. Malik, for example, wishes he had a more rewarding social life. Before he married Amy, he regularly played poker with his buddies and belonged to a cycling club. He thinks of that time as a period he felt "connected" and physically in good shape. He gave up these activities because he felt that being away from Amy would not be good for their relationship. He realizes that his thinking around that may not be accurate and that, in fact, meaningful friendships and fitness not only aid his well-being but have the potential to do the same for his marriage. The four-cell cost–benefit analysis form can be helpful here. Each cell includes the cost or benefit of approach or avoidance behavior (see Table 7.3). For example, have the patient identify the cost of avoiding fear. Malik is constantly distracted while he worries, and he feels like he is missing out on life. On the other hand, avoidance makes him feel temporarily better. After completing the form, ask the patient to weigh the pros and cons of these two strategies and what his or her goal is going forward. This exercise can enhance motivation for giving up avoidance and adopting an approach stance to life—becoming a "yes man."

Table 7.3 Cost–Benefit Analysis Form

Goal	Cost	Benefit
Avoid Fear: Worry and safety behavior use	• Distracted and never in the moment • Don't feel connected • Worry and safety behavior use are time consuming • Missing out on life • Wife is annoyed with my avoidance and safety behavior use • May be actually causing what I fear most; relationship difficulties and divorce	• I am prepared for or prevent potential catastrophes • Brief anxiety relief • Not away from my wife • Always know what my wife is doing
Approach Fun: Poker with friends and cycling club	• Away from my wife more • Won't know what my wife is doing • I'll be anxious	• Have fun • Be my ideal self • Get fit • Have more energy • Be more present with my wife

7.4.5. Common Pitfalls When Targeting Fears of Thoughts

(1) *The patient presents a new worry each session.* As depicted in Figure 7.5, patients who present with GAD frequently bring up new worries each session. It's important as a clinician to not get distracted or sidetracked by these new concerns. The evaluation has helped you identify the core themes that underlie many of these worries, and you can relay this to the patient, helping him or her understand that what emerges at surface may appear different yet is driven by the underlying core fears that you have discussed with him or her. Be sure to stick with one imaginal exposure at a time. Also, setting an agenda each session can help eliminate extra time that can easily be filled by the latest (and what feel like different) problems.

(2) *The patient reports that he or she is unable to vividly imagine the exposure.* If you and the patient are confident that the script should be working but the images are just not vivid, it may be helpful to have the patient practice vivid imagery. Consider the following exercise:

> Close your eyes and imagine a lemon. Imagine you can see the vivid yellow color. You can see the rough surface and feel it in your hand. Squeeze it slightly and see that it is ripe and gives a bit. Now imagine cutting into the lemon and seeing the juice mist out. Smell the mist. You can

feel your mouth water. Now squeeze the lemon juice into a spoon and place it in your mouth noticing immediately the sour flavor.

This exercise can help the patient see that his or her ability to imagine is better than he or she thought, and perhaps he or she can help you make the script even more vivid.

(3) *The patient is not showing within-session reduction in SUDs.* One reason this happens is the patient simply has not had enough time with the exposure. Nevertheless, keep an eye out for subtle safety behaviors and actions that send threat messages to the brain. For example, a patient may grip his or her chair tightly while recounting a trauma. We would ask the patient on the next trial to try it differently, with relaxed arms. Similarly, the patient may make fearful facial expressions during the imaginal exposure. Accordingly, we ask him or her to relax his or her facial muscles on the next trial.

7.5. Treating Fears of Images in OCD

Angela is a 29-year-old new mother, who works part-time as a paralegal. She describes her marriage to her husband Adrian as "wonderful," lining up with what she dreamed of as a child. They met and dated in college, married at 26, and moved to a small city where they started a law practice. Assisting her husband on most mornings of the week, Angela is heavily involved in the local community, mostly through church-related events (e.g., foodbank, Welcome Wagon, neighborhood cookouts, etc.) and other charities. Much of her life today mirrors that of her mom's when she was her age, and she feels proud of the fact that she has achieved that. Growing up, Angela was told that it's important to give more than you take. She attended Catholic school and joined her parents and extended family on a number of national and international mission trips in her teenage years. She describes these experiences as rewarding and as having shaped her values and the selection of activities that she finds meaningful today. She remembers first starting to be bothered by intrusive thoughts and images when she entered middle school. Prompted usually by conversations among her peers during recess, she would have what she experienced as disturbing sexual images and have difficulty turning them off. These intrusive images would cause her to feel guilty ("I felt like I was a bad person for having these") and be up late at night saying repeated prayers. Confession always helped, but these initial "experiences" with images set the stage for Angela to become warier of her own cognitive content. She started avoiding cues (e.g., conversations, music, media, movies) that could prompt disturbing images and immersed herself in activities that she felt could neutralize the feeling that she was a bad person. "Hanging on," Angela's fears of images became overwhelming and started interfering with her life when Sofia was born six months ago. Two days after coming home from the hospital, Angela picked up Sofia to feed her and was struck with the image of throwing her down the stairs. The imagery about hurting her baby expanded to include suffocation, stabbing, and drowning. Overwhelmed by these recurring images and her interpretation (e.g., "What if I actually end up doing this"; "I am a bad person"), Angela has developed a repertoire of safety behaviors, including avoidance (e.g., hired a full-time nanny, refrains from holding Sofia, removed sharp objects from the house), compulsions (e.g., prayer, replacing feared images with positive images), and reassurance seeking (e.g., asking Adrian whether she's is a bad person). As evidenced by a Yale–Brown Obsessive Compulsive Scale (Y-BOCS) score of 27 (see Chapter 9), she's debilitated by fear and avoidance and the resulting symptoms of depression (Patient Health Questionnaire 9 score is 12; see Chapter 9).

The case of Angela is characteristic of what we often see in patients with OCD, namely a person who presents with core fears—in this case harming someone and being a bad person—that diametrically oppose her values and the outcomes others associate with her. For this and other reasons, we find it's helpful to patients if we describe OCD in the third person—a "bully" that follows patients around and keeps an eye out for images the patients consider off limits. The bully tries to convince him or her that these images have great significance—thinking/imagining something disturbing is as bad as doing it or will cause it to actually happen (i.e., thought–action fusion). A patient's first natural reaction may be to argue with the bully or take steps to avert the catastrophe by engaging in "neutralizing" actions (i.e., compulsions or rituals). Ultimately, we want the patient to ignore the bully entirely. When the bully threatens Angela, we want her to do nothing. However, this can be difficult at first given a lifetime of arguing and finally giving into the bully. Thus, at first we ask Angela to allow the OCD bully to yell, scream, and do whatever it wants while doing nothing to prevent catastrophes, thereby simply acknowledging that she is experiencing false instead of true alarms. This initial phase of treatment is focused on threat disconfirmation, that is, regardless of the response, the image will not lead to catastrophic outcomes. However, the OCD bully is extra mean and will argue convincingly that there is no way to fully disconfirm the threats. This dialogue characteristic of OCD (i.e., the bully questioning logic as well as the compelling evidence of safety at hand) generates doubt (i.e., "I don't know that it is OCD"; "What if I am really a bad person?"). We have found that, rather than continuing the emphasis on threat disconfirmation, patients with OCD ultimately benefit from a shift to focusing on increasing comfort with uncertainty and doubt. Accordingly, we suggest making two modifications to planning and implementing exposure therapy when targeting the fears of images in OCD:

(1) education about the nature of obsessions and compulsions, and
(2) enhancing cognitive flexibility

7.5.1. Education about the Nature of Obsessions and Compulsions

Helping the patient understand what maintains the senseless cycle of internal experiences and corresponding neutralizing actions, it's helpful to precede exposure practice with specific education about obsessions and compulsions, how they are related, and how these are maintained over time.

> First let's take some time and define what we mean by obsessions, compulsions, and OCD. An obsession is a recurrent thought or image that is distressing. You may have heard the word used differently before now. The word *obsessed* is used for many different meanings in popular culture. For example, people will say they are obsessed with a hobby. In this case, they mean they like the hobby. However, obsessions are unwanted or intrusive thoughts. Others may say they are obsessed with their performance on an important test or interview so they need to prepare. Here, they mean they cannot stop thinking about a realistic situation. However, when we use the word *obsession* we mean not being able to stop thinking about something unrealistic like getting HIV from a doorknob. Typical obsession categories include harm obsessions (like harming yourself or others), contamination obsessions (by bodily fluids, germs, or chemicals), sexual obsessions (forbidden sexual thoughts or incest), hoarding obsessions (thoughts about acquiring and saving of unnecessary items), religious obsessions (blasphemy or morality), and symmetry/exactness obsessions. Like you, many people try to push away these aversive thoughts and images. This can be difficult. What often happens when you try to stop thinking about something? You usually end up thinking about it more. If I were to ask you to do anything you want but just don't picture a pink elephant over my head, what do you think would happen? You would think about it more. Not surprisingly, many people try other methods to neutralize or reduce the obsessions and the distress that comes with them. This is where compulsions come in. Compulsions (or rituals) are repetitive behaviors or mental acts people perform to alleviate distress from obsessions. For example, a child may have intrusive curse words that keep coming into his mind and he is frightened this means he will yell them aloud and that yelling them aloud will lead to dire consequences. He smacks his head

> in desperation repeatedly. The distress dissipates over time, and he learns that hitting his head is associated with a decrease in anxiety from the obsession. Over time, this action can become almost automatic. This is just one example of how a ritual can get linked to anxiety reduction from an obsession. Typical compulsion categories include cleaning/washing compulsions (hand washing, showering, house cleaning), checking compulsions (stoves, appliances, locks), repeating compulsions (rereading, rewriting), counting compulsions, ordering/arranging compulsions, and hoarding/collecting compulsions. Once these obsessions and compulsions become time-consuming and distressing and interfere with life and activities a lot, a person can meet diagnostic criteria for OCD."

As we discussed in Chapter 3, self-monitoring of thoughts, symptoms, and behaviors during the initial phase of treatment allows for the patient to see a personalized record of the cue–image–fear–compulsion relation, aiding the socialization to exposure therapy.

> I would like for you to start seeing your OCD, just like I do, like a phobia of images. We all know people with phobias. Consider my aunt: She will do whatever she can to avoid dogs. Although she knows that almost all dogs are friendly, she always feels sure that they will get her when she sees one. Like it's different in that moment, and all the logic goes out the door when she is in that moment. Why is she afraid of dogs? Because she acts in ways that signal danger: She makes sure that's she's prepared, as in she scans her surroundings, and she will flee when she sees a dog. These defensive actions send a strong signal of danger, as why else would she be doing that? Now consider your defensive actions. I know that you rely on them; they make you feel safe. But, they come at the same cost as they do for my aunt; that is, they keep the fear cycle alive. I'd like for both of us to see how this fear cycle plays out for you during the week. So, I am going to ask you to record your thoughts and defensive actions right after you experience intrusive images over the next week. I also think it's helpful if you kept track of cues or the factors other than seeing Sofia that evoke the images. My hope is that a week of data helps us to (a) further clarify the relation between obsessions and compulsions; (b) see the phobia; and (c) identify possible other fear themes or avoidance strategies that we should target in treatment.

7.5.2. Enhancing Cognitive Flexibility

In the processing of exposure practice, we initially start asking Angela if her predicted outcome actually occurred.

> You just repeatedly imagined the scenario of stabbing Sofia while you stood next to her crib holding a pair of scissors for the past 20 minutes. And, importantly, you didn't engage in any rituals in an attempt to feel safer. Did you end up harming her? Convince me that you are a bad person because of that. What do you make of the threat you attach to this image?"

Some patients benefit from this explicit focus on threat disconfirmation and as result experience a shift in their appraisal of harm: "Gosh that was intense that image, but you're right an image is just an image, like a movie is just movie." However, for some patients, especially those who experience doubt reinforced by the OCD bully, engaging in an exercise of logic can have paradoxical effects. That is, by challenging their faulty appraisals, which, in turn, are challenged by the bully (and so on), these patients end up increasing rather than decreasing the significance they place on their own cognitive content (i.e., "I keep talking about the image, so it must be important"). This is a trap in the treatment of fears of thoughts and images—when a patient finds it challenging to recognize that his or her concerns are indeed senseless (i.e., overvalued ideation) and complete disconfirmation is impossible (i.e., we cannot guarantee the outcome will not occur), you end up talking in circles. Rather than continuing to stress restructuring or reappraisal, processing with these patients can focus on enhancing cognitive flexibility. Consider the following specific learning objectives:

(1) *Learning to recognize we are not good at making predictions.* Review with a patient the predictions they have made in other domains (e.g., school, work, family politics, sports, the lives of family members/friends) to simply highlight that these have often been inaccurate, suggesting that attending to predictions may not prove to be worthwhile.
(2) *Learning to recognize the double standard.* If cognitive content is as significant as the patient argues it is, why is it that he or she doesn't focus more on images (and thoughts) of positive outcomes. Consider a homework assignment involving repeatedly imagining buying a winning lottery ticket and the effect it will have on his or her life.
(3) *Learning to tolerate uncertainty.* Feeling prepared and knowing what to expect can feel good, but is it necessary for a good outcome? Review with the patient his or her or others' experiences with positive surprises in life. These, by definition, were outcomes that came out of the blue and demonstrate that uncertainty does not have to be associated with negative outcomes per se. Also, highlight the patient's effective handling of uncertainty in many areas in her life. Ask the patient, for example, to call her husband to ask him if he lost his job that day. If the patient looks surprised by the request or tells you that's very unlikely, ask her, "How do you know?" Lastly, consider

revising the script for the imaginal exposure to center the feared outcome on uncertainty (i.e., having to live in the state of never knowing).

Changing a patient's relationship with his or her own cognitive content is at the heart of exposure therapy. Attaining cognitive flexibility (in addition to or instead of cognitive reappraisal) reflected by achieving one or more of the previously discussed learning objectives represents such a shift. Importantly, it is fully in line with the aim to build new memories of safety; that is, cognitive flexibility implies that thoughts, images, and memories are, indeed, safe.

7.5.3. Common Pitfalls When Targeting Fears of Images

(1) *The patient uses exposure as a ritual.* There is the potential for any activity done in an obsessional context to become ritualized. That is, instead of being a procedure for the learning of safety, the patient comes to view the exposure as a neutralization response—as a sort of talisman that, if executed correctly, will neutralize danger. For example, after many repetitions, the patient now may feel anxiety if he or she does not do an exposure in response to an obsession. Or the patient may feel the need to do the exposure exactly correctly. In these cases, we suggest the patient do the exposure "incorrectly." At this point, we suggest the patient try doing nothing when he or she has an obsession rather than exposure. We remind the patient that the goal is to become comfortable with discomfort rather than always trying to reduce discomfort.

(2) *The patient is reluctant because he or she argues that the proposed content for the exposure exercise is "not normal."* It's true that repeatedly listening to a script describing the scenario of Angela stabbing her baby Sofia is not normal. It's also not normal for a germ phobic to repeatedly jump in a dumpster or to repeatedly touch a public toilet seat without engaging in neutralizing rituals. Why do it then? The answer is because we want to overwhelm the patient's brain with information that he or she is safe. Yes, the patient preference is to be careful and not push the envelope (i.e., "I would rather not risk it"). We know, however, that the OCD bully latches on to complacency, thus interfering with fear extinction, allowing for the OCD to persevere.

(3) *The patient undoes ritual prevention.* It's a success when you have been able to complete exposure practice ensuring that the patient doesn't engage in neutralizing behaviors. The challenge often is to also ensure that the patient persists over time following the session. Like a smoker who made a quit attempt but lapsed at the end of the day following a fight with his spouse, the patient with OCD who has confronted the feared cue will be faced with the urge to neutralize in the hours following the exposure practice. If you cannot be available (by text or phone) yourself, we recommend

that you and the patient enlist the help of others who can check in and help the patient stay "abstinent." Consider the following instruction:

> Once we begin exposure, it's critical that you cease your compulsions. Every time you neutralize, you signal threat, keeping the fear cycle alive. Although it is difficult, it is also exciting to finally begin relearning safety around these uncomfortable thoughts and feelings in response to these images. I want you to plan for how you are going to resist your compulsions after the session. Please call or text me if you feel you are about to engage in a ritual and need some help staying the course. Alternatively, do you think we can enlist Adrian to hold you accountable and support you while you go through this part of the therapy?
>
> Now what to do if you end up engaging in a ritual, perhaps even without thinking about it? Of course, that can happen. If it does, let's agree to the rule that you: (a) Record it on your self-monitoring form and (b) immediately redo the exposure as we did it here. We call that "spoiling" the ritual.

(4) *The patient employs excessive reassurance seeking.* Directed by the OCD bully, some patients have difficulty engaging in practice and will stop asking questions like, "Is this safe? Am I doing this right?" Consider the following response to help the patient eliminate this maladaptive safety behavior.

> I understand you wanting to check on this or seek reassurance. It's the doubt that is part of OCD. It's the OCD bully directing you. We need to work together to start ignoring the bully, motivating him to direct his efforts elsewhere away from you. So, while I care for you and am tempted to answer each time you ask me to help you resolve your doubt, I know that doing so is a disservice to you. So, today I will answer that question, but I will not answer such questions in future sessions, helping you learn to relate to doubt differently, that is, doing nothing."

7.6. Treating Fears of Memories in PTSD

Daniela is a 22-year-old single female college student. Approximately one year ago, she stopped at a rest stop at around 5 AM. After using the restroom, she turned around to find a stranger with a knife demanding she remain silent. Over the period of the next hour she would endure brutal torture. As dawn light shown through the window, the rapist left the bathroom stall but told her he would be back and to stay in the stall. After several hours crouched in the corner, she summoned the courage to emerge from the restroom. She managed to drive herself to home and went straight to the shower. After showering she got in bed and hid under the covers, terrified. Over the past year, she dropped out of school and moved home to be with her parents and rarely ventures outside. Her life as she knew it ceased to exist. Her parents contacted the clinic to get her help after trying several medications and other clinicians.

From a small town, she was raised in a loving home with a commitment to strength and excellence reflected by her many academic and competitive sports achievements. Her family encouraged mental toughness and pushing away negative thoughts. She previously believed her future was bright with a degree, good job, marriage, and a family in store. Daniela is now shocked at her inability to cope with the rape and terrified by a drastic change in her world view. She feels weak for the first time in her life and that the world is now a dangerous, almost foreign place and she has no hope for a future. She assumes that a trauma such as hers is best left in the past and tries to distract herself from the memory and avoid other reminders (e.g., being home alone, men, colognes). Talking about it with her previous clinicians has only brought pain and terror. After each session, she would drink alcohol to help her sleep. She doesn't understand how exposure therapy would help. She is already being exposed to the memory daily with intrusive thoughts/images even though she tries to push it away. She is understandably skeptical about even seeing another clinician.

While growing up, Daniela learned to push away negative thoughts and images and that this would lead to mental toughness and strength. In many cases, this led to greater focus during academic and competitive sports. Not surprisingly, this was her go-to strategy to cope with intrusive and aversive memories of the trauma. The trauma memory became the enemy. The memory was dangerous and something to be avoided. However, the harder she tried to push it away, the more it seemed to enter her mind. Her inability to effectively control the memory made her think she was weak. Determined to make the strategy work she adopted behaviors to further attempt to push away the reminders by using distraction, avoiding things that reminded her of the trauma, and drinking alcohol. She first tried watching TV but quickly realized there were trauma reminders in the media (e.g. violent shows, crime stories). After much trial and error, she found that the only task that worked at all was to play solitaire on her computer and smart phone at home constantly with the blinds drawn. By shutting herself off from the world and playing solitaire she was often able to spend some time not thinking about the trauma. Her next challenge was sleep. Only alcohol helped her fall asleep. But then she would wake up in the middle of the night several times, and in the morning the memories returned and she would go right back to the solitaire. The constant use of her safety behaviors further strengthened the thoughts that the memory and world are dangerous and she was weak and unable to cope. Although her safety behaviors offered temporary relief, they also kept the symptoms going.

7.6.1. Recovering from Trauma

Trauma is relatively common and often results in immediate symptoms such as re-experiencing (e.g., intrusive memories, flashbacks, nightmares), avoidance of situations and trauma reminders, changes in cognition and mood (e.g. thoughts that the world is dangers, inability to cope, depression), and hypervigilance (e.g., angry outbursts, increased startle response, insomnia). Over time, most people naturally recover. However, for a substantial minority, these symptoms persist indefinitely without intervention. These individuals have developed a fear of the trauma memory and present in our clinics with PTSD. They can benefit greatly from exposure therapy that targets the fear of that memory. We recommend a few modifications to planning and delivering exposure therapy for the general outline provided in the first section of this chapter:

(1) education about the nature and treatment of PTSD,
(2) imaginal exposure involving the recounting of the trauma memory, and
(3) processing focused on the meaning of the trauma and trauma reactions.

7.6.2. Education about the Nature and Treatment of PTSD

Starting exposure therapy for PTSD is easier once you have helped the patient see that it's not the trauma that is the target but the fear of the trauma. Consider the following script:

> Before we start treatment, I would like to talk a bit about trauma reactions and how this treatment works. I want to start by talking with you about what we know often happens after a horrific event like the one you experienced. We know that most Americans will experience a trauma at some point in their lives. Most people that experience a trauma have some amount of intrusive memories, flashbacks, nightmares, avoidance of trauma reminders, thoughts that the world is dangerous, and a feeling of being on guard. For many trauma survivors, these symptoms decline over time. However, for others, they continue. Researchers investigated what makes symptoms continue like this. The difference appears to be pushing away the trauma memory and avoiding other reminders. Avoidance may be a natural reaction after a trauma, but in the long run it can keep the symptoms going. That is why in this treatment we will target avoidance by using

two methods to help you confront trauma-related thoughts and situations. First, we will use imaginal exposure to the trauma memory. The trauma you experienced was truly dangerous, but the memory of it is not, even though thinking about it is so distressing. We will do this together in the session in a systematic way that we know is therapeutic. After each imaginal exposure, we will talk about what your experiences were while doing the exposure and the meaning of the trauma more generally. We will work to make sense of a senseless situation. Imaginal exposure to the trauma memory helps you control the memory rather than the memory controlling you. Second, we will use in vivo (or in real-life) gradual exposure to other trauma reminders that continue to bother you. We will prioritize reintroducing those things you used to do and enjoy but that you have avoided since the trauma. Finally, another factor that maintains PTSD is the presence of unhelpful thoughts and beliefs. For example, most people we work with have thoughts that the world is now more dangerous and that they feel unable to cope. We will address these thoughts and help you get a more accurate view of the world and yourself. The take-away message today is that there is hope. This is a first-line treatment for trauma and has been studied in many studies around the world with approximately 85% of patients getting better.

7.6.3. Imaginal Exposure to the Trauma Memory

Imaginal exposure applied in the treatment of PTSD involves repeatedly recounting the trauma memory, which starts with the following rationale.

To help you recover from the traumatic event, I will ask you to revisit the trauma memory here with me today. If you notice, I am careful to use the word "revisit" not "relive." This is because I am not actually asking you to relive the trauma. Instead, I will ask you to recount or retell the trauma memory. I cannot emphasize enough that I recognize that the trauma was dangerous, but I know that the memory of it is not.

Imaginal exposure to the trauma memory will help you in several important ways. First, repeated exposure to the trauma memory will help differentiate the memory from the actual event. In this way, you are not retraumatized but learn that the memory of the trauma is just that—a memory. The memory will never become a "good" memory, but you will get so that you can think about it without a fear response; it will take the emotion out of it. Think of a frightening horror film that you may have seen more than once. The first time you saw it you likely experienced significant fear while watching it. However, when you watched it again it didn't seem nearly as frightening. What do you think would happen if you watched it over and over? Eventually the fear would go away, and it might even seem boring.

Second, repeated exposure to the memory will help you organize the memory. We find that initially the memory seems to have pieces missing and is not a smooth coherent story with a beginning middle and end. This organization and elaboration will help you see more clearly what exactly happened and file it away with your other memories. A trauma memory is unlike others. We can think of our memories as if they are organized into files. For example, you have a memory file for "going to a restaurant." When you eat out, you don't spend a lot of time thinking through what to do when you arrive. Even if it is a new place, you have a sense of what is about to happen. There will likely be a hostess, he or she will seat you and hand you a menu, you will order, get your food, eat, and then pay. You even have memory files for unusual things. If it snows in the summer, this would seem extremely unusual but would nicely fit into the ever-growing file of "weird things happen and I don't know why." However, a trauma memory has no file. In addition, a trauma memory has huge emotional content. We as humans have a drive to process and figure out our life events, particularly emotional ones. Until the trauma is processed, it is considered unfinished business and will keep intruding, begging for our attention. If you don't deal with the trauma memory, the trauma memory will deal with you.

Third, becoming comfortable with the memory often generalizes to other trauma reminders making your recovery more efficient. Because imaginal exposure is so important and central to this treatment, we will do it together in the sessions. I will ask you to recount the memory in a specific way—a way that may seem strange at first. I will ask you to close your eyes and recount the memory aloud in the first-person and present tense. I will give you a brief example of what this sounds like: So I'm driving on the highway at about 60 miles per hour. It is near sunset and the sky looks purple. I feel the air conditioning hitting my face, and I'm listening to a radio news station. I look into the rear-view mirror, and I see a truck coming up behind me quickly. Just then I see the traffic in front of me stopped. I slam on the brakes. I can feel a rush of adrenalin and tingles in my arms. I can feel I have pressed the brake to the floor, and I smell rubber from other cars who stopped suddenly in front of me .... And so on. Does this make sense? Before we start, we need to pick a starting and ending point. I want you to start the story at the last point you still felt safe before the trauma and end at the first point you felt safe again after the trauma. Finally, I will ask you for your SUDs just before we begin, every five minutes after that, and then again when we are done. While you are telling the story, I will only say, "What is your rating now?" You can just give me a number and then continue on. If you finish the memory and we still have time, we will repeat it as many times as we can.

Next, you can work together with the patient to complete an exposure planning worksheet (see Box 7.1). Ask the patient what he or she is most afraid will happen if he or she confronts the memory with imaginal exposure. In many cases,

Box 7.1 Daniela's Exposure Planning Checklist

Patient: *Daniela* **Date:** *09-06-2018*

Target threat appraisals (use response from the Posttraumatic Cognitions Inventory [PTCI]):

Feared outcome: *the memory will make me go crazy* Rating: *80%*

Feared outcome: *fear will peak and never go away* Rating:

Feared outcome: Rating:

Feared outcome: Rating:

Goals

Confront the memory repeatedly (imaginal exposure) and stick with it while doing nothing to manage her fear

Trauma memory items to include

- ❑ Starting Point: *walking into the restroom*
- ❑ Ending Point: *getting under the covers at home after a shower*
- ❑ Sights: *dark outside with some moonlight*
- ❑ Smells: *men's cologne*
- ❑ Tastes:
- ❑ Sounds: *rapist breathing and saying, "Say you love me"*
- ❑ Temperature: *hot and humid*
- ❑ Feelings/Emotions: *intense fear*
- ❑ Bodily Sensations: *stomach pain and nausea*
- ❑ Other cue(s):

Safety Behaviors: (plan when to fade/eliminate)

- ❑ Distraction: *playing solitaire*
- ❑ Food/drink: *limiting water intake to avoid public restrooms*
- ❑ Medications: *alprazolam*
- ❑ Cognitive rituals/lucky sayings (list):
- ❑ Social errors/mishaps (specify):
- ❑ Body posture during imaginal (e.g., curling up, covering face, facial tension): *clutching stomach*
- ❑ Voice (speaking quickly, slowly or in a quiet voice):
- ❑ Other:

Set specific and achievable behavioral goal (based on goals and manipulations above):

45 to 60 minutes of imaginal exposure in the office, learning into the feelings (e.g., giving up avoidance strategies) and allowing fear to run its course.

patients will say they are afraid they will unable to handle the exposure. For some this means it will make them go crazy or they will die. For others, they anticipate their fear will rise to an intolerable level and never go away. The goal is to test these hypotheses and revisit them after the exposure. Once you have discussed the patient's understanding of this information and answered any questions, conduct the imaginal exposure with the patient for approximately 20 minutes. At the end of the imaginal exposure, ask for a SUDs rating, saying something like, "Great job, open your eyes. You showed tremendous courage doing that. What was it like for you?" This is the beginning of processing the imaginal exposure.

7.6.4. Processing Is Focused on the Meaning of the Trauma and Trauma Reactions

The goal during processing is to guide the patient in making sense of the trauma memory and the meaning of the trauma in a more general sense. There is no right way to make sense of a trauma so you can ask questions and use active listening to try to understand his or her experience both while recounting the memory and in general since the trauma. Your goal is to understand the thoughts and feelings surrounding the trauma: What is it like to be him or her? Common questions we ask include:

- What was that like for you?
- What did it feel like physically to recount the trauma?
- What did it feel like emotionally to recount the trauma?
- What was it like compared to what you expected?
- What do you think your life would have been like without the trauma?
- How is your life different now because of the trauma?
- How do you think your life will be different going forward because of the trauma?

Patients frequently describe their life on a particular trajectory before the trauma, and after the trauma life veered onto an entirely different trajectory. You can explore how the patient sees these two very different lives. The new life may, at first, appear entirely negative to the patient. Over time, however, patients often add more realistic and even positive aspects. For example, they may find that they no longer take life for granted. You can also share your own observations as a clinician. For example, you can point out any trends in SUDs before, during, and after the exposure. If there is not a reduction in SUDs, then you can tell the patient that (a) he or she demonstrated great courage in continuing despite high anxiety and (b) nothing catastrophic happened (i.e., he or she was anxious but experienced no harm).

7.6.5. In Vivo Exposure to Trauma Cues and Avoided Situations

We also integrate in vivo exposure to treat PTSD. In vivo exposure targets real-life trauma reminders and activities the patient used to enjoy but now avoids since the trauma. Consider the following script for introducing in vivo exposure.

> Next, let's talk about situations you used to enjoy but avoid since the trauma. We will make a list of these situations together and talk about how to re-engage in these activities in a therapeutic way so that you can enjoy them again. First, let's discuss the rationale for this exercise. Last session we discussed how some avoidance of situations, people, places, and other trauma reminders is a natural reaction immediately following a trauma. Although the avoidance alleviates anxiety in the short-run, it can keep the symptoms going in the long-run. Exposure in vivo will help your symptoms in several important ways. First, you have developed a habit of reducing anxiety through escape and avoidance. Confronting your fears one at a time will break this habit and eventually start to generalize to other difficult situations. Second, when you repeatedly enter your feared situations and nothing bad happens, you will learn that they are safe again. Third, some trauma survivors believe that if they stay in the feared situations their fear will either never go away or that it may just keep getting higher and higher. By staying in the situation for a prolonged period of time, they learn that the fear always eventually goes away. Finally, by confronting your fears successfully, you will regain a sense that you are strong and able to cope with anxiety. We can expect that when you confront a feared cue in a gradual, systematic, prolonged, and repeated manner, the fear will always eventually go away.

Once the notion of in vivo exposure has been discussed, we move to creating items on the hierarchy. Although the items on the hierarchy can be anything that the patient now fears due to the trauma, the most valuable items are those that represent valued activities that have been blocked by PTSD-related avoidance. That is, we prioritize items that the patient previously enjoyed but now does not do because of the trauma. Here we are trying to simultaneously expose them to feared cues to reduce their fear and conduct behavioral activation for any depressed mood. For each item we have them estimate what their fear would be if they confronted the cue right now (see Table 7.4).

After generating 5 to 20 items, we place them in order (a sorted Excel sheet can be helpful here). For homework, we want the patient to choose an item on the

Table 7.4 Daniela's In Vivo Hierarchy

	Situation	SUDs
1	Going to a movie with friends	60
2	Going to a movie alone	90
3	Looking at a cartoon picture of a pocket knife	55
4	Looking at a picture of an actual pocket knife	65
5	Looking at a real pocket knife	85
6	Holding a real pocket knife	100
7	Going to a public restroom alone	90

Note. SUDs = Subjective Units of Distress Scale.

hierarchy he or she can make the focus of initial practice. We want the patient to select an item that is difficult enough that if he or she conquered it, it would feel good. However, we do not want the patient to select an item so difficult that he or she will not follow through on the homework. For many patients with other anxiety disorders, this corresponds roughly to a 60 or 70 on the fear scale. One additional consideration is to select an item that can be practiced daily. For example, although an international flight may be a great exposure someday, this cannot be practiced every day. For the first exposure, we recommend the patient only completes the single assigned item each day. The patient and clinician can decide together at the next session to repeat the same in vivo exposure or to move on following the guidelines described in Section 7.2.4.

7.6.6. Subsequent Sessions

Subsequent sessions roughly follow the same structure. During these sessions you can decide to trim some of the recounting of the memory to be more efficient. For example, you may notice the patient reports very low SUDs during the beginning and end of the imaginal exposure. In this case you can discuss with the patient trimming the beginning and end to focus on the more activating parts of the trauma. In addition, in later sessions we further trim the memory to just the most activating part. Edna Foa has termed this phase "imaginal exposure to Hot Spots." In these sessions you will also continue to modify the in vivo exposure homework.

7.6.7. Pitfalls When Targeting the Fears of Trauma Memories

(1) *Overengagement and dissociation.* Some patients may become overly engaged in the memory or dissociate during the imaginal exposure. Indications of overengagement include uncontrollable crying, trembling, or even getting up and leaving the room. Indications of dissociation can include extremely long pauses, getting lost in where the patient is in the story. In these cases, we tell patients that we want them to keep one foot in the memory and one foot here in the room with us (i.e., effective learning of safety requires the ability to discriminate between the past true alarm of the trauma and the current false alarm of *memories* of the trauma). Interventions can include having the patient tell the memory with his or her eyes open, using the past tense, or even writing the trauma out on paper or while typing. Using grounding techniques can further halt dissociation. For example, you can pause and ask the patient to stand up, rub his or her hands together, and describe the weather outside (to ground the patient in the present).

(2) *Underengagement.* Very low fear ratings may suggest underengagement. It is helpful to add additional sensory details to the script in this case. We can ask the patient during the imaginal what he or she sees, hears, smells, and feels. We also want to make sure the patient is not leaving out important parts of the trauma or being careful how he or she talks about the trauma. For example, some patients are reticent to curse or use slang. Sometimes they are embarrassed in front of the clinician to include such details or more natural language for them (or at least the language they used during the trauma). You can probe to make sure this is not happening and encourage the patient to use whatever language that is consistent with the way the memory unfolds in his or her mind without filtering it.

(3) *Multiple traumas.* Many patients have experienced multiple traumas that cause distress. As part of the intake, we make sure to begin with the trauma that causes the most current distress or re-experiencing symptoms. If imaginal exposure reduces the fear entirely to one trauma and there remain re-experiencing symptoms from another trauma, imaginal exposure can also be conducted to the untreated trauma. We typically find that imaginal exposure to one to three total traumas generalizes to others. However, we should only work on one trauma at a time.

(4) *Relationship with a perpetrator.* If the patient is still in a relationship with an abuser, we wait to initiate imaginal exposure until this relationship is

terminated. Otherwise, the trauma is likely still ongoing, and the environment is not safe for the patient.

(5) *What are safe in vivo exposures?* At times, the patient and clinician cannot be sure what exactly are safe in vivo exposure exercises. For example, the clinician may not know if walking to the store in the patient's neighborhood is safe. Likewise, the patient may no longer feel able to determine what is considered safe behavior. To address this concern, we will often ask the patient to use the behavior of others as a guide. In the patient's neighborhood, is it customary to walk to the store during the day? Do most other people in the neighborhood consider this safe? Did the patient consider this behavior safe before the trauma? The answer to these questions can help determine if the proposed in vivo exposure is safe.

(6) *Symptom exacerbation.* It's not uncommon for symptoms to get worse before they get better. This is because the patient has been avoiding the trauma memory and reminders. Once he or she begins to confront these reminders, anxiety frequently rises before it falls. Research shows, however, that this pattern of symptoms is not cause for alarm. Patients who get worse at first and those that show a steady decline in symptoms from the beginning get equally better.

(7) *Patients who believe but are not sure they were abused as a child.* Imaginal exposure therapy is contraindicated for patients who do not have a clear memory of a trauma with a beginning, middle, and an end.

(8) *Complex PTSD.* Complex PTSD is prolonged repeated exposure to trauma (sex trafficking, long-term domestic violence, concentration camps, etc.). Exposure therapy can be effective with this population, but it is not designed to specifically address the additional symptoms that may be present in complex PTSD (e.g., emotion dysregulation, distorted perceptions of perpetrators). Additional treatment may be needed to address the added interpersonal difficulties that come with complex PTSD. We often use a phased approach with complex PTSD. This begins with emotional stabilization followed later by exposure therapy if PTSD is present.

(9) *The patient refuses to repeat the trauma memory in the first imaginal exposure.* Many patients may initially refuse to repeat the imaginal exposure after the first trial. We always encourage patients to repeat the imaginal exposure to assure they are not sensitized. However, some patients still refuse. In this case, we can encourage them to at least listen to the recording with us. If they still refuse, we ask them to practice listening to the recording for homework and that we will repeat the imaginal exposure

at the next session but will go through it multiple times. Eventually, most patients are able to withstand multiple trials within session.

7.7. Conclusions

In this chapter, we discussed the treatment of internal threats including thoughts, images, and trauma memories. Imaginal exposure is particularly effective for the treatment of these fears. It has advantages over in vivo exposure because it can be used when in vivo exposure may not be appropriate or feasible (e.g., for combat traumas, fear of contracting a disease or dying alone or harming someone). It can be used alone or in combination with in vivo exposure. When used in combination, it is generally delivered first in therapy (sequentially) or along with in vivo exposure (concurrently). Imaginal exposure therapy steps include identifying the core threat (downward arrow technique) or trauma memory, developing an imaginal exposure script/planning sheet, delivery of imaginal exposure, processing of the imaginal exposure (what was learned/meaning), and assigning home practice (listen to recording daily). Imaginal exposure can be used as a transdiagnostic approach to reduce fear. However, we discussed slight modifications in the cases of GAD, OCD, and PTSD.

8
Combining Exposure Therapy with Medications

8.1. Overview

When recovering from any disorder characterized by anxiety and avoidance, return to full functioning means that, eventually, one successfully returns to once-avoided situations and events. Yet, under conditions of partial response, patients may have less anxiety but continue to have the disability associated with ongoing avoidance. This is often the profile of symptoms for partial responders to medication, where anxiety may be improved, but there is enough anticipatory anxiety and fear in phobic situations to maintain avoidance and hamper full functioning. These are often the patients referred for combination treatment after having been treated with psychopharmacology alone for months or years. In this chapter, we consider three situations where combination treatment is encountered:

(1) when patients come to psychosocial treatment already on medications;
(2) when medications are initiated at the same time that exposure therapy is initiated; and
(3) when exposure therapy is initiated for the goal of medication discontinuation.

8.2. Treating Patients Already Taking Medication

It's common for patients who have achieved a partial treatment response with pharmacotherapy and who wish to continue with their medication to be referred for add-on psychosocial treatment. There is good news for such referrals; failures to respond adequately to pharmacologic treatment do not predict difficulties responding to exposure-based treatment. Patients taking medication for anxiety have an excellent chance to achieve additional treatment gains with exposure-based treatment. Nonetheless, ongoing medication treatment does introduce several issues for both the efficacy and staying power of exposure. These issues include both

(1) the attribution of treatment gains to medication, and
(2) context effects.

The core feature of both of these issues is that ongoing medication use makes the safety learning from exposure therapy conditional—conditional on the presence of medication. For example, research shows that if patients undergoing combination treatment attribute their treatment benefits to medication rather than cognitive-behavioral treatment, they face higher rates of relapse when medications are discontinued. These attributions are not the only predictor of relapse. Pharmacologic treatment also provides a unique context for safety learning due to both "pill-taking "and the "feel" of taking medication (an internal context). Due to these unique contexts, patients may learn safety only in the presence of these cues. To make these issues clear, let's return to the learning node model from previous chapters. Figure 8.1 depicts safety learning outside the context of medication for a particular phobic cue. Figure 8.2 depicts similar safety learning, but in the context medications. Note that medication use is linked to cognitive attributions ("I am better on medications"), the daily physical act of pill-taking, and the feel of being on medication. All three of these features

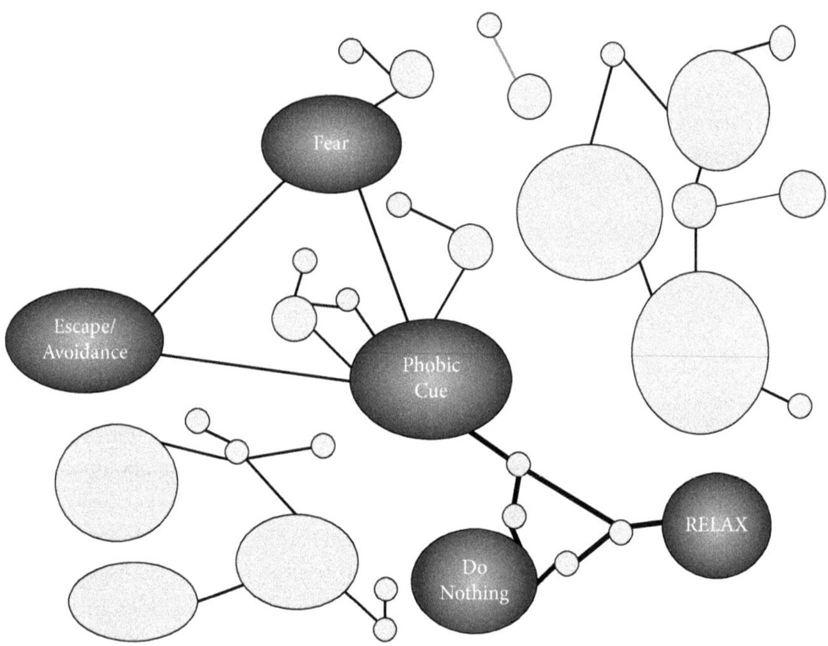

Figure 8.1 Memory node model reflecting safety learning outside the context of medication use.

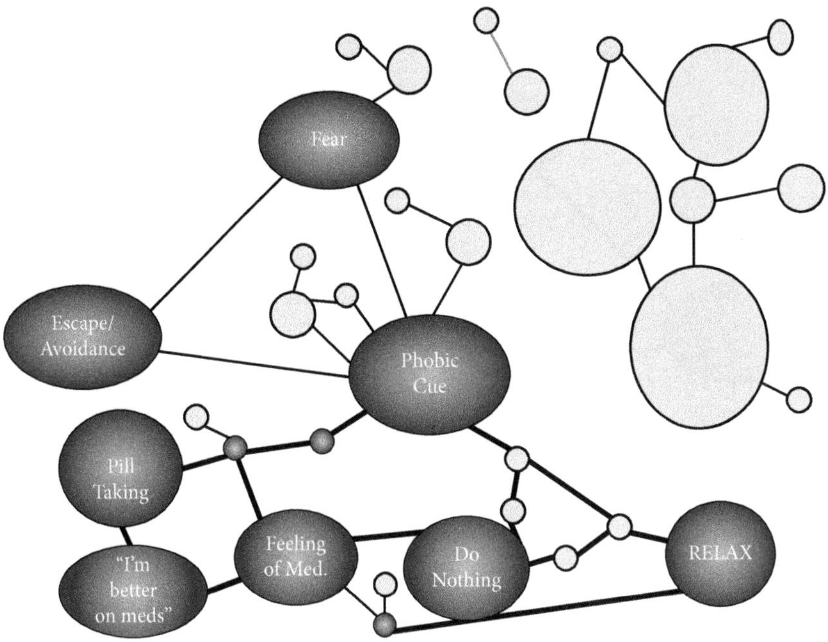

Figure 8.2 Memory node model reflecting the specificity of safety learning in the context of medication use.

may be important to maximize the benefits of exposure-based treatment. And when the context changes with medication discontinuation, safety learning may be attenuated, as depicted in Figure 8.3.

The management of the first of these factors—attributions of treatment gain—is aided by close monitoring of symptoms, so that the patient can link objective symptom levels to the elements of treatment being provided. For patients already on medication, this means that providing feedback on symptom levels needs to be made particularly salient before beginning exposure therapy: "This is your level of symptoms when taking medications, before starting exposure therapy." Weekly monitoring thereafter (see Chapter 4) should be part of each session's content, with the clinician explicitly asking the patient for his or her attributions about further reductions in symptoms achieved in psychosocial treatment.

A crucial part of this strategy is that all medications need to be taken on a fixed daily dose, so that medications are an *unvarying backdrop* to the addition of exposure therapy. This fixed dose recommendation especially includes benzodiazepine medications. For this medication class (prominently including alprazolam, clonazepam, and lorazepam), it will be important for the psychosocial

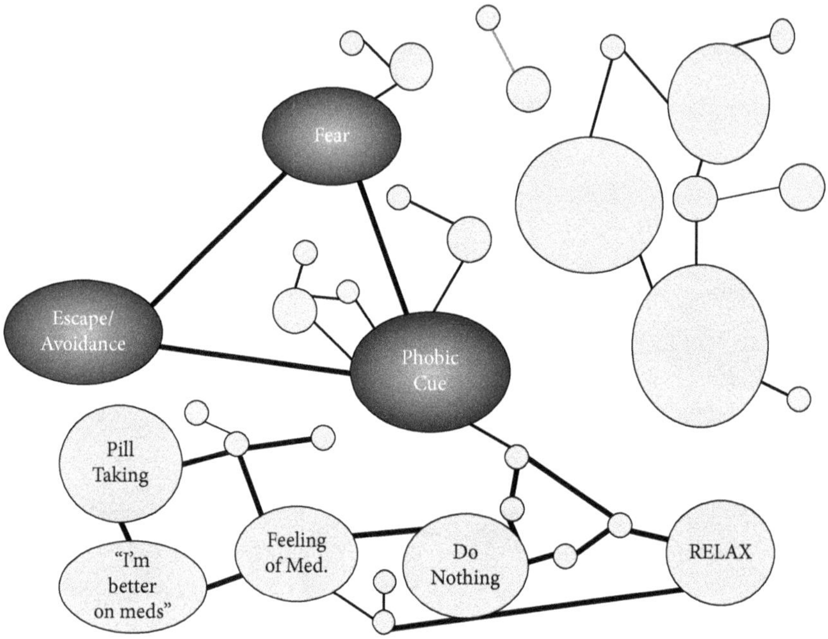

Figure 8.3 Memory node model showing relapse (return of fear) due to dependence of safety learning on the context of medication use.

clinician to working with the prescribing clinician to eliminate "as needed" (or "prn") dosing during the weeks of exposure therapy. Such prn dosing seriously clouds the attribution of treatment gains to anything other than the effects of the last pill taken. Nonetheless, patients may rightfully conclude from their symptom monitoring that subsequent treatment gains may be dependent on a backdrop of medication use to help exposure therapy work ("I could never have entered those situations without using my medications"). This attribution is (a) difficult to challenge while the patient continues to take medication, and (b) likely places the patient at an enhanced risk for relapse should he or she discontinue taking his medication. In a restatement of the "What happens in Vegas stays in Vegas" saying, it appears that "What happens on medications stays on medications" is an apt way to conceptualize the conditional safety learned under combination treatment. In sum, patients who improve on the combination of exposure therapy and medication should maintain these gains well as long as they are maintained on medications. But if medication is later discontinued, patients face a context change and a threat to both their attributions and the learned context surrounding improvement. A proportion of these patients will respond to this context change with partial relapse.

What is done about this enhanced risk of relapse? Providing exposure-based treatment across a medication discontinuation phase provides the most obvious answer. In this way, patients are treated on medication, and subsequently this safety context of medication is faded while exposure therapy continues, helping the patient learn more unambiguous safety ("I can do it regardless of whether I take my medication"). Indeed, some pharmacologists prefer this approach, providing benzodiazepine medication in a brief treatment format, with referral to exposure therapy and fading of medication as the patient makes initial treatment gains with exposure. Except for cost and the potential for withdrawal symptoms (see the following discussion), this method is conceptually similar to initiating exposure therapy while patients have a host of safety behaviors (traveling with a cell phone, water, and antacids in the pocket) that are faded as the patient learns initial (conditional) safety in their phobic situations.

Yet, many patients will not be ready to discontinue their medication during the current phase of treatment. For patients making this choice, we emphasize the importance of reinitiating exposure therapy whenever the patient does want to try a medication taper. This scenario is more common with use of antidepressant medications (prominently including escitalopram, fluoxetine, fluvoxamine, paroxetine, and sertraline), where treatment guidelines recommend continuation treatment for at least six months once treatment is initiated.

8.3. The Simultaneous Initiation of Combination Treatment

We avoid this scenario whenever possible. That is, all of the previously discussed issues—attribution of treatment gains and context effects—are intensified when treatments are initiated together. If possible, we would prefer to be in the lead with psychosocial treatment, avoiding the complexities of co-occurring medication treatment, except when nonresponse results. However, this may not be what the patient desires. When both treatments are initiated together, we make it clear that the patient may not know which gains are from which treatment. Nonetheless, prn dosing should be expressly avoided to reduce the magnitude of this issue. Ultimately, for these patients, we believe that reinitiation of exposure therapy before, during, and after medication taper will be necessary to enhance retention of treatment gains.

8.4. Referrals for Help with Medication Discontinuation

The use of exposure therapy as an aid to medication discontinuation involves three issues:

(1) treating residual symptoms,
(2) treating the re-emergence of a disorder as medication efficacy fades, and
(3) treating withdrawal symptoms.

Treating residual symptoms of anxiety is the most straightforward process, consistent with all previous chapters, but with one additional caveat: Patients referred for medication discontinuation may be relatively comfortable with the current level of symptoms. This means that exposure therapy will involve moving them from a level of relative comfort through a temporary anxiety phase on the road to even greater comfort. This caveat is also apt for the treatment of re-emerging symptoms and medication withdrawal symptoms. In short, patients referred for medication discontinuation do not enter treatment with the same motivational force of high symptom levels. Instead, their motivation is linked to a desire for medication-free status. Because of this, we believe extra care needs to be taken to helping them become more comfortable with their experience of anxiety prior to exposure. In other words, exposure to symptoms (Chapter 5) should be a prelude to other exposure, as guided by their particular profile of concerns about symptoms. Interoceptive exposure is also the core strategy for helping patients effectively tolerate the withdrawal symptoms that may emerge from taper of their medications. That is, regardless of whether the treatment target is the re-emergence of symptoms in the context of exposure to avoided situations, or the biological induction of symptoms due to medication withdrawal, developing a sense of *safety with symptoms* is the right prescription (as per Chapter 5).

For the goal of aiding successful medication discontinuation, skills for tolerating symptoms are developed and rehearsed in the context of interoceptive exposure and are later applied to the challenges of medication taper. Specifically, with interoceptive exposure, patients learn the skills of "relaxing with a sensation and doing nothing to manage it." Patients subsequently are asked to recall and apply these skills during the otherwise unique conditions of medication withdrawal. The emergence of withdrawal symptoms is common for taper/discontinuation of benzodiazepine medications, but withdrawal symptoms have also been documented for some antidepressants (e.g., the shorter half-life serotonin-selective antidepressants like paroxetine) if a slow taper is not used. In the following sections, we detail procedures for benzodiazepine discontinuation because this is the more challenging process. Readers should consider these same procedures for taper and discontinuation of antidepressants but can anticipate that this process is much easier than what is detailed for benzodiazepine medications.

To clarify the nature of our approach, let's turn to examples where preparing patients for the evocation of symptoms is a central task. Consider treatment for those rare events that are likely to engender high anxiety but for which regular exposure cannot be easily arranged: Events such as the high test anxiety experienced by people when taking crucial life-transition tests like the GRE, LSAT, or MCAT. Certainly, low-intensity exposures can be arranged with practice tests, but for some test-anxious individuals, these practice tests can be too easily discounted as "not like the real thing," and it is only the "real thing" that provokes a strong anxiety response. As such, the task for the clinician is not to try to eliminate anxiety to the high-stakes test but to ensure better performance on the test despite the presence of anxiety. Specifically, interoceptive exposure is used to reduce the disruptive power of anxiety by having the patient both study and take practice tests while experiencing anxiety symptoms induced by interoceptive exposure. The goal is to aid the development of an effective cognitive focus while experiencing anxiety sensations and then *transfer* this skill to the high-stakes testing conditions. This follows the classic behavioral principle that effective transfer of a newly learned skill to a new situation depends in part on the shared cues between the conditions where the skill was first learned and the conditions where it is to be used. Interoceptive exposure during studying and practice tests provides these shared internal cues.

We use similar strategies for lawyers anxious about rare and high-stakes court appearances. Again, exposure in the context of mock courtroom presentations may be viewed by patients as "not real enough" or "without the dire consequences of 'blowing it' in court." Accordingly, we have lawyers present their brief in the context of induced sensations of anxiety to learn that they can present well under these internal circumstances. Subsequently, anxiety may be cued in their "high-stakes" presentation but is more tolerable and does not escalate because the anxiety-about-anxiety response has been treated by the pre-exposures. Feelings of confidence arise in knowing one can present competently despite the presence of anxiety.

Returning to the issue of managing medication withdrawal symptoms, the goal of pretraining is to establish a sense of safety with symptoms prior to their induction from the medication taper. That is, during pretraining, patients have the opportunity to sample and learn to react differently to symptoms that are induced over the course of minutes prior to the emergence of taper-related symptoms that may last for hours or days. This change in timeframe deserves additional attention. Many exacerbations in anxiety and panic are often short-lived and situational dependent. This is not the case with withdrawal symptoms, which may be prominent for hours to days as the patient's body adapts to the absence of a given dose of benzodiazepines. If symptoms become too continuous, the patient and his or her physician can slow the taper to give a break from symptoms during the period between dosage reductions. Nonetheless, during taper, patients are in need of a frame for coping with symptoms that are more chronic than what is commonly rehearsed in interoceptive exposure.

One very useful frame is that of coping during a cold or flu. All of us have experience coping with the symptoms of a cold or flu over several days and are often able to pursue role demands (e.g., going to work, taking care of children) despite these ongoing symptoms. And typically, people have no anxiety response to these symptoms even though the symptoms can be quite strong. Moreover, some of the symptoms of benzodiazepine withdrawal—headaches, body aches, odd taste in the mouth, etc.—are the same as those associated with a flu (see Figure 8.4). Consequently, a model for effective coping is to have patients frame their withdrawal symptoms in a context of coping with the "benzodiazepine flu." In terms of the memory-node model from Chapter 2, symptoms induced from interoceptive exposure can be considered in the frame of long-standing skills in coping with the flu.

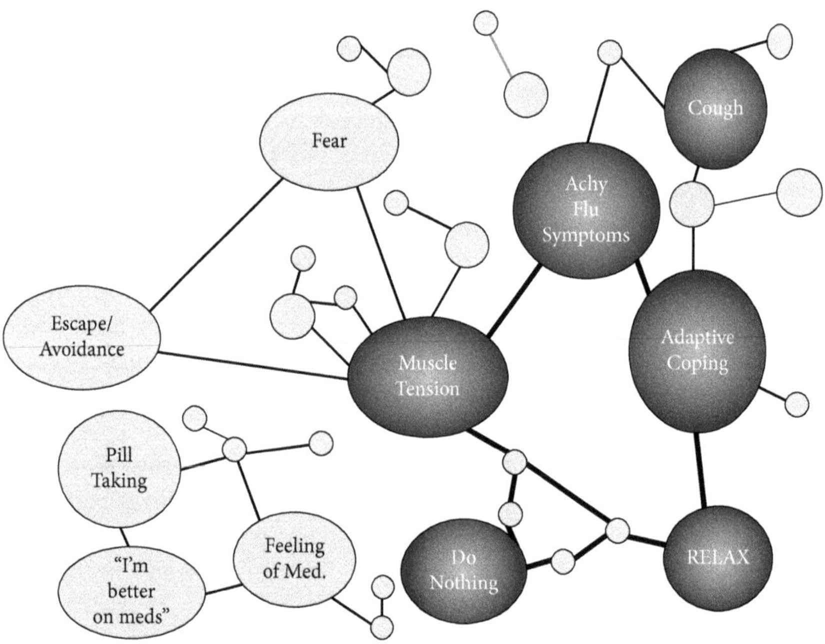

Figure 8.4 The benzodiazepine flu model for coping with tension, represented as memory nodes.

In addition to the value of pretraining before the initiation of taper, ongoing sessions with interoceptive exposure enable the clinician to check in on symptoms from the taper and to rehearse coping with these symptoms in an exposure model—increasing the intensity of these symptoms with interoceptive exposure and rehearsing: (a) doing nothing with the symptoms and (b) a benzodiazepine flu frame for coping. That is, to increase comfort with benzodiazepine withdrawal symptoms, it is helpful to give the patient ongoing reminders of their coping skills (doing nothing to manage the symptoms and relaxing with them as per Chapter 5) in focused sessions with the clinician. These ongoing interoceptive exposure sessions also provide patients with preparation for any return of symptoms they may experience during their transition to psychosocial treatment from their previous medication treatment.

Box 8.1 lists some of the prominent symptoms of benzodiazepine withdrawal. Patients will differ on the time-course of symptom emergence as well as which symptoms will emerge. Some guidance, nonetheless, is provided by knowledge of the half-life of the benzodiazepine under taper: The longer the half-life of the agent, the slower the clearance of the drug and, hence, the greater the delay of symptom emergence. Table 8.1 provides information on common benzodiazepines, the relative potency of these agents (in equivalent dosages to alprazolam), and the half-life of these agents. Considering two particularly common agents—alprazolam and clonazepam—clonazepam tends to be more potent than alprazolam (1 mg clonazepam would be providing approximately the same effects as 1–2 mg of alprazolam), and the effects of these doses would last approximately twice as long for clonazepam than alprazolam given the longer half-life for clonazepam. These effects are evident in clinical taper

Box 8.1 Common Symptoms of Benzodiazepine Withdrawal

Anxiety
Irritability
Insomnia
Muscle tension
Headache
Sweating
Shaking hands
Nausea
Difficulties concentrating
Perceptual distortions
Metallic taste in mouth

Table 8.1 Characteristics of Common Benzodiazepines

Drug	Dose Equivalent (mg)	Approximate Half-Life in Hours
Alprazolam	1.0	12–15
Clonazepam	0.5	15–50
Lorazepam	2.0	10–20
Diazepam	10.0	20–100

scenarios. For example, in our studies, we saw later emergence of withdrawal symptoms for patients taking clonazepam (half-life 15 to 50 hours) than those taking alprazolam (half-life 12 to 15 hours). Indeed, it is not uncommon to observe patients undergoing alprazolam taper experiencing a surge of symptoms weekly, after every reduction in their dose. In contrast, some patients taking clonazepam would make it to the end of taper with very few symptoms, only to have symptoms surge dramatically several days after the final dose. Regardless of the profile of symptom emergence, patients needed pretraining with coping with symptoms to weather these symptom challenges across the medication taper weeks.

The actual medication taper is done in collaboration with the prescriber to pick a slow taper appropriate to the patient and his or her goals for being medication free. Overall, the target is a taper rate that is safe and attenuates the strongest of withdrawal symptoms, yet does not keep the patient focused on tapering for a prolonged period of time. For example, one recommended taper slows the rate of taper as the patient gets to lower doses. Specifically, as represented in alprazolam equivalent doses (see Table 8.1), we have used a rate of 0.25 mg reduction every two days for doses above 2 mg, and a slowed rate (0.25 mg reduction every four days) for doses of 2.0 mg or less. For clonazepam, this schedule translates to 0.25 mg reduction every four days for doses above 1.0 mg, and 0.25 mg every eight days for doses 1.0 mg and below.

8.5. The Case of Steve

To put together the elements of treatment, let's consider the case of Steve. Steve is a 34-year-old man who has been taking benzodiazepines for his panic disorder for seven years, after a somewhat prototypic onset of panic disorder in his mid-20s. He takes 2 mg of clonazepam a day, 1 mg in the morning and 1mg in the late afternoon, to try to control any breakthrough symptoms that may occur with waning medication effects from once-a-day dosing. His panic disorder has been moderately managed by his clonazepam use, where he now has only one mild panic episode per week, down from an early history of daily panic attacks. Yet, his life remains tightly circumscribed to his safe situations. He can travel almost anywhere when his wife or best friend is with him (among his friends, only his best friend knows of his panic disorder), but he does not drive beyond a several-mile radius alone, paying particular attention to staying off roads and driving times where he may feel trapped by traffic jams. Steve's case represents a classic challenge in that panic disorder almost universally ensures attention to and fears of somatic symptoms of anxiety. These fears sometimes intensify with partial response to benzodiazepine treatment, because of the way each dose of medication gives relief from anticipatory anxiety or panic symptoms that otherwise appear uncontrollable; these are the feared symptoms that are likely to be evoked during benzodiazepine taper. Figure 8.5 provides a model of his fears of symptoms.

One of the first interventions for Steve was to discuss the importance of no prn medication use during his new treatment, staying with the fixed dose of 1 mg in the morning and 1 mg in the evening. Steve was asked to discuss this with his prescriber as a prelude to a direct discussion between his psychosocial clinician and his prescribing clinician about Steve's goals, the taper schedule, and the type of treatment to be provided. His prescriber recommended a slow taper of

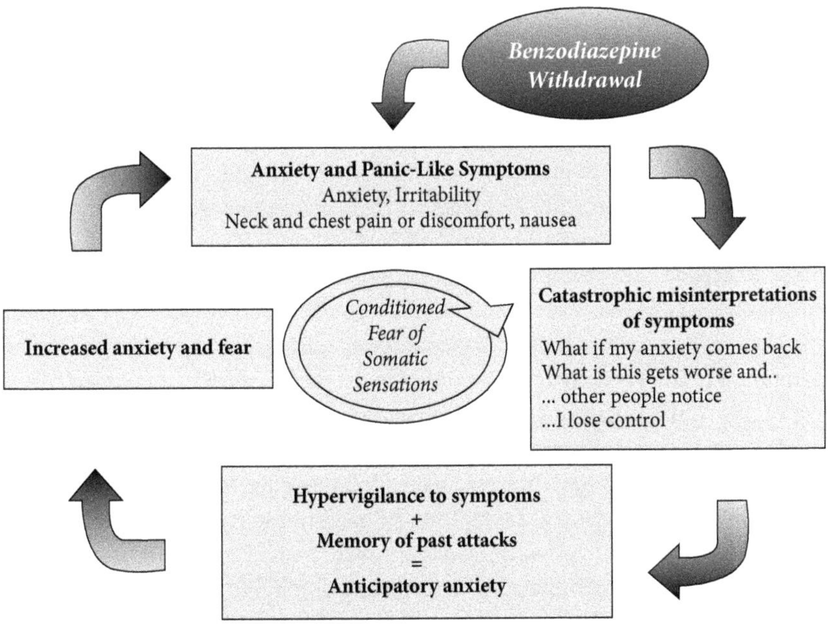

Figure 8.5 Understanding Steve's fears of symptoms.

0.25 every four days until he was down to 1 mg, and then 0.25 every week until he successfully discontinued his medication. Thus, his taper was targeted to take just over six weeks. However, this taper was not to start for a month to allow exposure therapy to provide the pretraining to change Steve's relationship with the symptoms that were likely to be induced by the taper.

During this preparatory period, Steve was given a model for treatment, his fears in relation to symptoms were discussed, and a program of interoceptive exposure was started following procedures outlined in Chapter 5. With each exposure, the clinician had Steve rehearse relaxing with the sensations and noticing that despite the presence of symptoms he could feel relatively comfortable. Home practice was initiated, and Steve chose to practice symptoms with his partner for the first two weeks. This led Steve to be able to increase the intensity of the symptoms rapidly, having his partner practice along with him and discuss how they could get comfortable with odd sensations, including remembering other times they were comfortable with sensations such as dizziness and disorientation and how these sensations were similar to those induced at drinking parties they attended together in college. Once initial comfort with a range of symptoms was established, the clinician had Steve start inducing symptoms when he was alone at the house or alone in the car in his own driveway. Then, as the week of the initiation of the medication taper drew near, the clinician introduced the benzodiazepine flu model and completed interoceptive exposure while rehearsing this frame for relaxing with the symptoms. The clinician also had Steve conduct interoceptive exposure and then go about role activities (imagined or actual) while feeling the symptoms and accepting them.

Steve's preparation of the skill of relaxing with the symptoms continued untested until the second week of taper. At that point, Steve began to experience not only an increase in general anxiety but also a metallic taste in his mouth, an increase in neck tension, and nausea. These symptoms would fade as he got to the fourth day of taper and then would resurge with his next dose reduction. Steve discussed these symptoms with his physician, and together they decided to continue the taper at the identified rate. The clinician continued a program of rehearsing relaxing with the benzodiazepine flu, using an intensification of symptoms in interoceptive exposure as a model for practicing acceptance-based coping. Steve did not have a further worsening of symptoms until the last 0.5 mg of his taper. During this time, he extended the taper by an additional week to "give himself a breather." It took him two weeks following the last dose to finally feel fully "normal"—at the level of symptoms he had prior to the medication taper.

With the goal of benzodiazepine discontinuation achieved, Steve is now in an excellent position to eliminate his remaining agoraphobic avoidance. His taper-related symptoms have given him a wealth of confidence in his ability to respond differently to symptoms. He is now primed to apply these skills to situational exposure practice, where he will approach situations ready to accept symptoms until he becomes fully comfortable in the situations. In short, his fear-of-fear cycle has been largely treated, and he just needs to generalize these skills to his avoided situations. As per recommendations, in Chapter 5, the clinician links all driving/travel exposure to valued activities, so that the patient can attend to what he is achieving in a given situation other than simply tolerating anxiety. As a final stage in therapy, interoceptive exposure practice is conducted in the context of the stop-and-go of rush-hour traffic.

8.6. A Return to Considering Resilience

As is apparent, helping patients cope well with withdrawal symptoms makes rich use of the skills from Chapter 5. In that chapter, we discussed comfort with anxiety-related symptoms and sensations as a core feature of resilience. Research shows that relative comfort with the experience of anxiety-related symptoms (low anxiety sensitivity) predicts resilience in a wide range of situations ranging from persisting with goal behaviors like cutting down Internet use and quitting smoking to lower levels of mood-dependent eating or exercise avoidance. In this chapter, we further illustrated this general point by detailing how interoceptive exposure can be used to promote resilience to the symptoms that emerge as part of benzodiazepine discontinuation. Pretraining with interoceptive exposure was used to provide a patient with a frame for coping with the biologically driven symptoms of medication withdrawal. This same strategy can be applied to helping patient for other symptoms of withdrawal, such as the nicotine withdrawal linked to smoking cessation. The goal is to help smokers relax with these sensations, so that these nicotine withdrawal sensations do not push them back to tobacco use. We also noted that such preparation for future symptoms involves an active transfer of training. The coping response of "relaxing with symptoms" (or, relatedly, applying a "benzodiazepine flu" interpretive frame) was rehearsed in the context of interoceptive exposure practice, in preparation for application of these coping strategies in the context of benzodiazepine withdrawal symptoms.

We also discussed how a transfer of training approach can be used to increase resilience to rare and especially salient phobic events that may not readily lend themselves to situational exposure approaches. Our examples included test-anxious students taking the GRE or the courtroom-phobic lawyer facing a trial. Test-taking or public-speaking skills are practiced under conditions of interoceptive exposure, so that the symptoms induced by the high-stakes GRE or courtroom environment do not derail adaptive behavior in these contexts. Truth be told, we routinely recommend to our graduate students that rehearsals for their first professional talks should include interoceptive exposure. Knowing that you are able to give an effective talk while having anxiety symptoms provides very important learned safety. In all these applications, we are following the general rule:

> If the novelty or striking importance of a situation prevents situational exposure, use interoceptive exposure to create safety with the anxiety symptoms that may emerge, aiding resilience for novel performance demands.

Finally, in the context of discussing resilience training, it is always important to consider the range of procedures that can be used to enhance resilience to aversive sensations/emotions. For example, aerobic exercise naturally exposes individuals to a variety of arousal-related somatic symptoms: Rapid breathing, rapid heart rate, sweating, stomach upset, and a wide variety of aches and pains. Accordingly, exercise can be used as part of resilience training for related somatic sensations. We have shown that exercise can be used to reduce anxiety sensitivity relatively rapidly, and we have applied this skill to coping with nicotine withdrawal symptoms. This is a transfer of training skill that involves helping patients increase their exercise, note their resilience to sensations during exercise, and then apply this resilience skill to coping with nicotine withdrawal. Regular exercisers also get the benefit of a mood lift that is well documented for aerobic exercise. This mood lift alone can also improve resilience to subsequent symptoms.

9
Assessment Strategies

9.1. Overview

In this chapter, we provide a list and brief description of a selection of empirically supported self-report measures that can help you and the patient assess whether you're meeting the goals of exposure therapy. As such, this chapter complements Chapter 4, which discusses how clinicians can go about ascertaining success, and the chapters focusing on the implementation of exposure therapy, which emphasize the importance of assessment and make specific suggestions for how to integrate assessment in the session. Consistent with the book's structure and the approach we take to personalized exposure therapy, we have organized the list of measures by feared cue (i.e., emotions and related physical sensations, people, and thoughts, images, or traumatic memories) and domain (i.e., intervention targets such as appraisals and safety behaviors; outcome/symptoms).

9.2. Fear of Emotions and Related Physical Sensations

9.2.1. Intervention Targets

9.2.1.1. Anxiety Sensitivity Index (ASI-3)

- *Assesses*: Fear of anxiety and related sensations
- *Number of Items*: 18
- *Scoring*:
  - Rated on a 5-point scale ranging from zero (very little) to 4 (very much)
  - Scored by summing the item scores, with possible total scores ranging from zero to 72
- *Norms*: Based on research examining cut points for the ASI-3 that identify more at-risk individuals, we believe that intervening with interoceptive exposure is certainly important for those with scores above 23 and can be considered part of useful resilience training for anyone with scores above 17 (Allan, Korte, Capron, Raines, & Schmidt, 2014; Allan, Raines, et al., 2014; see Chapter 11).
- A copy of the measure can be obtained at http://www.anxietysensitivityindex.com

9.2.1.2. Distress Tolerance Scale (DTS)

- *Assesses*: Tolerance of emotional distress
- *Number of Items*: 15
- *Scoring*:
  - Rated on a 5-point scale ranging from 1 (strongly agree) to 5 (strongly disagree)
  - Scored by first reverse-scoring item 6 and then by averaging all item scores, with possible scores ranging from 1 to 5
- *Norms*: Mitchell, Riccardi, Keough, Timpano, and Schmidt (2013; see Chapter 11) have reported the following means (standard deviations) for different samples:
  - Diagnosis of primary anxiety disorder: 2.87 (0.89)
  - Nonclinical: 3.43 (0.83)
- A copy of the measure can be requested from Jeffrey Simon at Jeffrey.Simon@usd.edu

9.2.1.3. Panic Appraisal Inventory (PAI-I, II, III)

- *Assesses*: Fear of panic attacks
- *Number of Items*: 45
  - PAI-I (anticipated panic subscale)—15 Items
  - PAI-II (negative consequences subscale)—15 Items
  - PAI-III (coping self-efficacy subscale)—15 items
- *Scoring*:
  - Rated on a 0% to 100% scale, with percentages indicating the following per subscale:
    - PAI-I—% likelihood of having a panic attack
    - PAI-II—% strength of concern about consequence
    - PAI-III—% confidence to persist
  - Scored by averaging the item scores, with possible scores ranging from zero to 100
- *Norms*: Feske and Beurs (1997; see Chapter 11) have reported the following means (standard deviations) for individuals with panic disorder and agoraphobia:
  - PAI-I: 47.0 (20.8)
  - PAI-II: 45.5 (18.8)
  - PAI-III: 31.2 (17.3)
- A copy of the measure can be requested from Michael Telch at telch@austin.utexas.edu

9.2.1.4. Texas Safety Maneuver Questionnaire (TSMQ)

- *Assesses*: Use of safety behaviors to manage fear of panic attacks
- *Number of Items*: 50
- *Scoring*:
  - Rated on 5-point scale ranging from zero ("yes, but not to manage anxiety/panic") to 4 ("always")
  - Scored by summing the item scores, with possible total scores ranging from zero to 250
- *Norms*: Kamphuis and Telch (1998; see Chapter 11) have reported the following mean (standard deviation) for patients with panic disorder: 78.43 (33.95)
- A copy of the measure can be requested from Michael Telch at telch@austin.utexas.edu

9.2.2. Outcomes

9.2.2.1. Panic Disorder Symptom Severity Scale (PDSS)

- *Assesses*: Severity of panic disorder symptoms
- *Number of Items*: 7
- *Scoring*:
  - Rated on a 5-point scale ranging from zero (none) to 4 (extreme)
  - Scored by summing the item scores, with possible total scores ranging from zero to 28
- *Norms*: Shear et al. (1997; see Chapter 11) have reported the following mean (standard deviation) for individuals with panic disorder and mild or no agoraphobia: 11.13 (3.01)
  - Suggested cut-off score for remission: <5
- A copy of the measure can be obtained at http://www.goodmedicine.org.uk/files/panic,%20assessment%20pdss.pdf

9.3. Fear of People

9.3.1. Intervention Targets

9.3.1.1. Appraisal of Social Concerns (ASC)

- *Assesses:* Perceived threats in social situations
- *Number of Items*: 20
- *Scoring*:
  - Rated on a 100-point scale ranging from zero (not at all concerned) to 100 (extremely concerned)
  - Scored by averaging the item scores, with possible total scores ranging from zero to 100

- *Norms*: Telch et al. (2004; see Chapter 11) have reported the following mean (standard deviation) for individuals with social anxiety disorder: 45.41 (20.61)
- A copy of the measure can be requested from Michael Telch at telch@austin.utexas.edu

9.3.1.2. Subtle Avoidance Frequency Examination (SAFE)

- *Assesses*: Use of safety behaviors to manage the fear of social rejection
- *Number of Items*: 32
- *Scoring*:
  - Rated on a 5-point scale ranging from zero (never) to 4 (always)
  - Scored by summing the item scores, with possible total scores ranging from zero to 128
- *Norms:* Cuming et al. (2009; see Chapter 11) have reported the following mean (standard deviation) for individuals with social anxiety disorder: 49.9 (19.7)
- A copy of the measure can be obtained at https://www.mq.edu.au/research/research-centres-groups-and-facilities/healthy-people/centres/centre-for-emotional-health-ceh/resources

9.3.2. Outcomes

9.3.2.1. Liebowitz Social Anxiety Scale (LSAS)

- *Assesses*: Severity of social anxiety disorder symptoms
- *Number of Items*: 24
- *Scoring*:
  - Rated on a 4-point scale ranging from zero (never/none) to 3 (severe/usually)
  - Scored by summing the item scores, with possible total scores ranging from zero to 128
- *Norms*: Fresco et al. (2001; see Chapter 11) have reported the following means (standard deviations) for different samples:
  - Diagnosis of social anxiety disorder: 74.53 (23.31)
  - Nonclinical: 13.49 (12.70)
  - Suggested cut-off score for remission: <30
- A copy of the measure can be requested from Michael Liebowitz at mrliebowitz@yahoo.com

9.4. Fear of Thoughts, Images, and Trauma Memories

9.4.1. Intervention Targets

9.4.1.1. Anxious Thoughts Inventory (AnTI)

- *Assesses*: Anticipated social and health threats and worry about worry
- *Number of Items*: 22
- *Scoring*:
  - Rated on a 4-point scale ranging from ranging from zero (almost never) to 3 (almost always)
  - Scored by summing the item scores, with possible total scores ranging from zero to 88
- *Norms*: Wells (1994; see Chapter 11) has reported the following mean (standard deviation) for individuals with generalized anxiety disorder:
  - Social Worry: 24.0 (5.1)
  - Health Worry: 14.3 (3.6)
  - Meta Worry: 19.7 (3.9)
- A copy of the measure can be requested from Adrian Wells at adrian.wells@manchester.ac.uk

9.4.1.2. Intolerance of Uncertainty Scale (IUS)

- *Assesses*: Intolerance of uncertainty
- *Number of Items*: 12 items
- *Scoring*:
  - Rated on a 5-point scale ranging from 1 (not at all characteristic of me) to 5 (entirely characteristic of me)
  - Scored by summing the item scores, with possible total scores ranging from zero to 60
- *Norms*: Laposa, Collimore, Hawley, and Rector (2015; see Chapter 11) have reported the following mean (standard deviation) for individuals with an anxiety disorder: 37.21 (SD 10.35)
- A copy of the measure can be obtained at https://adobe99u.files.wordpress.com/2014/12/ius.pdf

9.4.1.3. Obsessive Beliefs Questionnaire-44 (OBQ-44)

- *Assesses*: Concerns about thoughts and images
- *Number of Items*: 44

- *Scoring*:
  - Rated on a 5-point scale ranging from 1 (disagree very much) to 7 (agree very much)
  - Scored by summing the item scores, with possible total scores ranging from 44 to 308
- *Norms*: The Obsessive Compulsive Cognitions Working Group (Obsessive Compulsive Cognitions Working Group, 2005; see Chapter 11) has reported the following means (standard deviation) for individuals with obsessive compulsive disorder: 174.3 (50.2)
- A copy of the measure can be obtained at https://iocdf.org/wp-content/uploads/2016/04/08-Obsessional-Beliefs-Questionnaire-OBQ-44.pdf

9.4.1.4. Thought–Action Fusion Scale (TAF)

- *Assesses*: Perceived threats associated with thoughts and images
- *Number of Items*: 19
- *Scoring*:
  - Rated on a 5-point scale ranging from zero (strongly disagree) to 4 (strongly agree)
  - Scored by summing the item scores, with possible total scores ranging from zero to 76
- *Norms*: Rassin, Merckelbach, Muris, and Schmidt (2001; see Chapter 11) reported the following means (standard deviations) for different samples:
  - Obsessive-compulsive disorder: 30.69 (14.64)
  - Other anxiety disorders: 28.29 (13.07)
- A copy of the measure can be requested from Jack Rachman rachman@mail.ubc.ca

9.4.1.5. Posttraumatic Cognitions Inventory (PTCI)

- *Assesses*: Perceived threats and other negative cognitions related to traumatic memories
- *Number of Items*: 36
- *Scoring*:
  - Rated on 7-point scale to indicate level of agreement, ranging from 1 (totally disagree) to 7 (totally agree)
  - Scored by summing the item scores, with possible total scores ranging from 36 to 252

- *Norms:* Foa, Ehlers, Clark, Tolin, and Orsillo (1999; see Chapter 11) have reported the following median score (standard deviation) for individuals with posttraumatic stress disorder: 133 (SD 44.17)
- A copy of the measure can be obtained at http://www.goodmedicine.org.uk/files/ptsd,%20assessment,%20pcti.pdf

9.4.2. Outcomes

9.4.2.1. GAD-7

- *Assesses*: Severity of anxiety symptoms
- *Number of Items*: 7
- *Scoring*:
  - Rated on 4-point scale ranging from zero (not at all) to 3 (nearly every day).
  - Scored by summing the item scores, with possible total scores ranging from zero to 21
- *Norms*: Donker, van Straten, Marks, and Cuijpers (2011; see Chapter 11) reported the following mean (standard deviation) for individuals with generalized anxiety disorder: 14.4 (SD 4.0)
  - Suggested cut-off score for remission: <5
- A copy of the measure can be obtained at https://www.integration.samhsa.gov/clinical-practice/gad708.19.08cartwright.pdf

9.4.2.2. Patient Health Questionnaire 9 (PHQ-9)

- *Assesses*: Severity of depression symptoms
- *Number of Items*: 9
- *Scoring*:
  - Rated on 4-point scale ranging from zero (not at all) to 3 (nearly every day).
  - Scored by summing the item scores, with possible total scores ranging from zero to 27
- *Norms*: Kroenke, Spitzer, and Williams (2001; see Chapter 11) reported the following cut-off score for major depressive disorder: 10
- A copy of the measure can be obtained at https://www.phqscreeners.com/sites/g/files/g10049256/f/201412/PHQ-9_English.pdf

9.4.2.3. Yale–Brown Obsessive Compulsive Scale (Y-BOCS)

- *Assesses*: Severity of obsessions and compulsions
- *Number of Items*: 10
- *Scoring*:
  - Rated on 5-point scale ranging from zero (none) to 4 (severe).
  - Scored by summing the item scores, with possible total scores ranging from zero to 40
- *Norms*: Rosario-Campos et al. (2006; see Chapter 11) have reported the following mean (standard deviation) for individuals with obsessive-compulsive disorder: 24.2 (6.9)
  - Suggested cut-off score for remission: <13
- A copy of the measure can be obtained at https://iocdf.org/wp-content/uploads/2016/04/04-Y-BOCS-w-Checklist.pdf

9.4.2.4. Posttraumatic Stress Diagnostic Scale (PDS-5)

- *Assesses*: Frequency/Severity of posttraumatic stress disorder symptoms
- *Number of Items*: 20
- *Scoring*:
  - The symptom items are rated on a 5-point scale of frequency and severity ranging from zero (not at all) to 4 (6 or more times a week/severe).
- *Norms:* Foa et al. (2016; see Chapter 11) have reported a score of 28 as a cut off for a probable posttraumatic stress disorder.
  - Suggested cut-off score for remission: <11
- A copy of the measure can be obtained at https://pdfs.semanticscholar.org/aacd/644f69bf38cccf4a7e84f244e8c3e18cee96.pdf

10

Psychoeducation about Anxiety, Fear, and the Role of Exposure

10.1. Overview

This chapter provides psychoeducation about the nature, causes, and exposure treatment of anxiety and related disorders in a patient-friendly format. The handout that follows can provide guidance in the first sessions as you socialize patients to treatment. We often describe to patients how common it is to have difficulties thinking clearly during episodes of high anxiety. Overlearning relevant material (including home review of therapy concepts) increases the chances it will be available even during such times. The goal is to make patients informed collaborators on the treatment of anxiety. Psychoeducation represents a first step. The text that follows in "handout" format is available on the companion website (www.oup.com/us/personalizedexposure).

10.2. The Alarm System: Worry, Anxiety, and Panic

Fear is designed to protect us and keep us safe. It motivates us. If it were not for anxiety and fear we would not show up to meetings on time or jump out of the way of an approaching car. Fear, when it happens in response to exposure to a real threat (i.e., true alarm), is very important for survival. However, if fear and anxiety are cued by things that do not actually pose significant physical threat/danger (i.e., false alarms; e.g., insects/animals, people, emotions, bodily sensations, images, thoughts, traumatic memories), these symptoms and associated avoidance can get in way of living. Thus, in exposure therapy we work to knock out false alarms that get in the way of achieving happiness.

10.3. Definitions: Stress, Worry, Anxiety, and Fear/Panic

What is the difference between stress, worry, anxiety, and fear/panic? *Stress* is best defined as the psychobiological reaction to demands. A demand is anything that takes mental space (good or bad). Examples include your job, family, friends, activities, a wedding, a death, or hobbies. The more demands and the larger they are, the more mental space they occupy (see Figure 10.1). Thus, either a lot of small demands or one single huge demand can cause significant stress. The total magnitude of all demands determines the amount of stress experienced.

When the body detects too many demands/stress, the natural biological drive/urge/reaction is to isolate and withdraw. This natural reaction can precipitate depression. To feel depressed at times is also normal. The problem is when people do not eventually re-enter the world and their activities, in which case the depressed mood can continue because of a lack of positive reinforcement. It should be noted that this is one way in which prolonged depressed mood emerges, but there are many more pathways to depression. People frequently ask if stress is harmful. The answer may surprise you. Acute or temporary stress actually improves your immune system. For chronic stress, however, it depends on how you *think* about or perceive stress. Many very busy people are stressed but do not suffer the negative consequences of chronic stress while others do. Some research shows that if you believe your stress is dangerous and extremely aversive, then you are at greater risk for health problems. However, if you feel that your

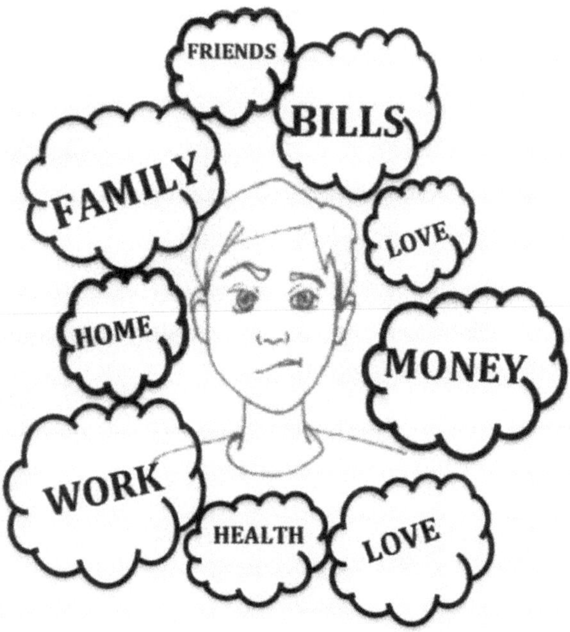

Figure 10.1 Stress as a function of demands.

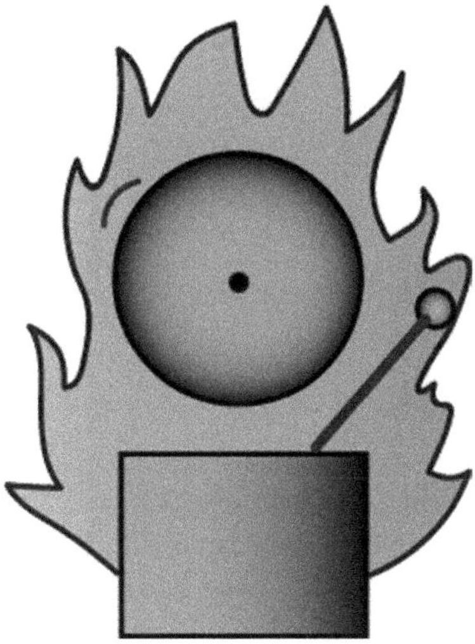

Figure 10.2 The human alarm system.

stress is a natural reaction to help you get through all the things you have going, then people do not suffer the same health problems.

Fear is different from stress and can be described as an alarm system. Fear is not unique to humans and most living things have some form of it. The alarm system is designed to keep us safe from danger much like a fire alarm (see Figure 10.2).

People could have designed actual fire alarms that include a nice green glow with a quiet pleasant soft voice that tells us, "Greetings all, a fire has been detected, please pursue safety at your leisure." In this case, many of us would ignore such a warning and keep working, assuming it was a false alarm. For this reason, fire alarms are wisely designed so that we are not capable of ignoring them—they drive even the most unflinching of us to leave the building. Your alarm system is designed the same way. It is designed to be annoying and uncomfortable so that it motivates us to fight or flee danger, and, importantly, like the fire alarm, it is also completely harmless in itself. Your alarm system is designed to be motivating but is itself completely safe.

In more advanced animals including humans, fear is can be conceptualized as being on a continuum including worry, anxiety, and panic. All humans worry, have anxiety, and panic or fear from time to time. The proximity of the threat determines where one is on the continuum (see Figure 10.3).

Worry is a response to perceived threats that are off in the distance (e.g., you are going camping in six months, and you hear there are venomous snakes in the woods). Worry is a verbal activity, which implies thinking in sentences such as

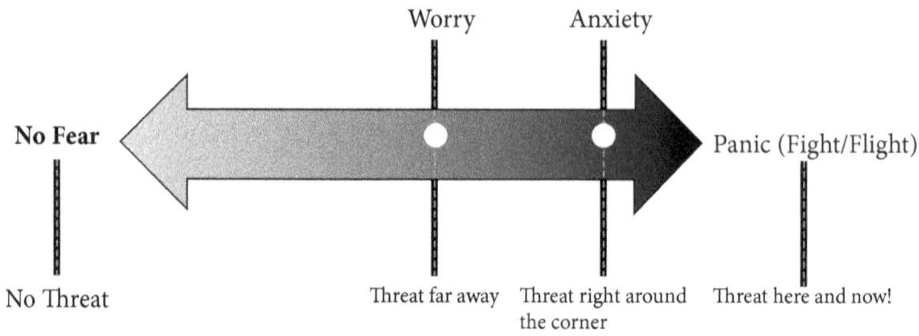

Figure 10.3 The fear continuum.

"Okay, so I have that camping trip in six months, and I am afraid a snake will bite me and I will die." This activity is associated with feelings of tension, being on edge and "nervous," but it does not activate your fight/flight system to the point where you see major increases in adrenalin and heart rate, etc. This worry part of the alarm system motivates you to prepare for things in the future but without activating the cascade of physiological responses seen later along the fear continuum. Also, given the threat is way off in the distance, behavioral inhibition or freezing is uncommon.

Anxiety occurs when the perceived threat is right around the corner. Using our camping example, you are now at the campsite and hear a rustling in the bushes. Given your concern, you will notice physical symptoms caused by nervous system activation like racing heart, sweaty palms, rapid breathing, shaking, nausea, and/or an urge to urinate. Anxiety prepares us to fight or flee at a moment's notice when the threat actually emerges. High anxiety can last for days.

Panic occurs when the perceived threat is here and now. You're at the campground, and a snake darts from the bushes toward your ankle. Panic can only last a short time; it comes on quickly and also dissipates in a short time. It motivates you to fight or flee immediately. The take-home message is that your alarm system is designed to protect you. It is designed to feel uncomfortable to motivate you to flee or fight in response to danger.

10.4. True versus False Alarms

It's important to make a distinction between a true alarm and a false alarm. A true alarm is useful because it occurs and when you perceive a threat that is real, whereas a false alarm is not useful because it occurs when you perceive a threat by mistake. For example, a sympathetic nervous system response is helpful and appropriate when you suddenly see a car headed toward you as you cross the street: It helps you get out of the way and avert harm. Having the same reaction when you notice an increase in heart rate, when you attend a party, when you experience an intrusive thought, or when you're reminded of a traumatic experience is not helpful; it just leaves you with excess "energy" as you will not use it to fight or flee from a threat because there is none. One job for your clinician is to help you redefine your fears into true alarms and false alarms and to help you develop a new approach for reacting to false alarms.

Our alarm system is set to err on the side of caution, to be sensitive to not miss danger/disease (more false positives than false negatives). That's why roughly 40% of people report having a panic attack at some point in their lives. You can see that it is appropriate to fight or flee when there is an actual danger. However, if there is no actual threat, then fighting or fleeing is not adaptive. The appropriate behavioral response to a false alarm is to do nothing and continue your current planned activity. Exposure therapy is about helping you become better at that and, by doing so, get rid of false alarms altogether.

10.5. Anxiety versus Anxiety Disorder

As previously discussed , worry, anxiety, and fear are designed to protect us and keep us safe. So, when do they become disorders? First, they must be false alarms: Worry, anxiety, and/or fear in response to relatively safe stimuli (fear of flying, fear of public speaking, etc.). Second, for the fear to be considered a disorder, it must interfere with the life and activities of the person a lot. Examples include not being able to leave the house for fear of having a panic attack, refusing to live on a ground floor or house due to a fear of spiders, missing meetings and deadlines and getting fired due to time-consuming obsessions and compulsions, getting a divorce over constant reassurance-seeking due to a fear of cheating, etc. The stimuli that are the focus of the fear helps determine the specific anxiety and related disorders.

10.6. Understanding Your Anxiety

In Table 10.1, we describe the impact of the body's alarm system (the sympathetic nervous system) on various bodily functions, the designed purpose for helping us, and, finally, the symptoms one may notice as a result. None of these effects are harmful to a healthy body, but they are designed to be annoying and motivating like the fire alarm to get us to act (even if we do not need to, as in the case of a false alarm).

Table 10.1 The Cause and Purpose of Symptoms You May Notice When Anxious or Panicking

Symptoms You May Notice	What Is the Cause and Purpose?
Physical System	
Heart racing and feeling like it is beating out of your chest	The heart beats faster (heart rate) and harder (stroke volume) to circulate oxygen to muscles in preparation for action. **Not Harmful**
Sweating	Perspiration to cool you off while you fight or flee. Some people also believe that sweating is designed to make you slippery to predators. Some sweating can also improve your grip (ever lick your finger to turn a page?). **Not Harmful**
Breathlessness, smothering sensations while breathing, and tremors/shaking	To prepare to fight and flee, muscles contract all over the body including between the ribs that makes expansion of the ribs outward difficult. **Not Harmful**
Lights become brighter	Pupils dilate to be able to see better at night. **Not Harmful**
Nausea, urinary urgency, and diarrhea	The body attempts to rid noncritical contents and weight. There is no purpose holding onto food, urine, or fecal matter during a life and death struggle. It will weigh you down. **Not Harmful**
Stomach pains and dry mouth	Digestion stops including saliva production. Again, there is no purpose digesting food now. All energy is diverted to fight/flight. **Not Harmful**
Elevated blood pressure	Blood vessels in the extremities constrict to pull blood from the extremities toward the vital organs. Also, constricted blood vessels in your arms and legs mean you bleed less if cut. **Not Harmful**
Lightheadedness	To take in more oxygen (O_2) and rid the body of carbon dioxide (CO_2) while fighting and fleeing, respiration rate increases. When your respiration rate increases due to sympathetic nervous system activation but you do not take action (not using the extra O_2 and not producing extra CO_2), the CO_2 level falls quicker than it is replenished resulting in a state called hypocapnia (low CO_2), which can lead to feeling lightheaded. These symptoms can also be produced by voluntary hyperventilation (rapid/deep breathing). **Not Harmful**
Blushing	Unlike blood vessels in extremities that constrict, some vessels such as in the face actually dilate in response to the sympathetic nervous system. **Not Harmful**

Table 10.1 Continued

Symptoms You May Notice	What Is the Cause and Purpose?
Mental System	
Difficulty concentrating	The sympathetic nervous system forces you to focus on the threat, not on other things. **Not Harmful**
Hypervigilance for threat when frightened	This forces you to search the environment for potential threats. This is meant to keep you on edge and prepared to react. **Not Harmful**
Behavioral System	
Avoidance	Avoidance is the primary response drive from anxiety. The best way to prevent a disaster is to avoid the dangerous situation altogether. **Not Harmful**
Urge to flee	The urge to flee is the primary response drive from panic. This is designed to get you away from the threat. **Not Harmful**

The take-home message from Table 10.1 is that your alarm system is designed to:

(1) protect you from danger, and
(2) create discomfort to motivate you to act.

Everyone has his or her own profile of symptoms that define his or her anxiety response. Some people sweat more, some people tremble more, and some people feel dizzy. Some people have a brief burst of anxiety when they confront something they fear; other people have their symptoms wax and wane over a longer period. As part of treatment, you and your clinician will get to know your particular profile of symptoms, and your clinician will help you react differently to these symptoms to meet your goals. One aspect of this profile includes how quickly your body turns off the alarm reaction. The body seeks balance (homeostasis), and there is an opposite system (the parasympathetic nervous system) that kicks in and reverses all the effects of the arousal/fight/flight (sympathetic nervous) system. The sympathetic nervous system cannot stay activated. Nor should it; an alarm system is only valuable if it turns on and off. A system that stays on has no value. After periods of arousal, the parasympathetic nervous system kicks in and calms things down, often leaving you tired after a strong anxiety/panic episode.

Whether you leave the frightening situation (avoidance/fleeing) or not, the parasympathetic nervous system will always return the system to rest/digest. Indeed, a principle of exposure therapy, staying in the frightening situation without doing anything, allows your parasympathetic nervous system to kick in and reduce your physiological response and fear eventually. Obviously people ask us, "How long does this take?" The answer is "It depends." Think of the alarm again like a fire alarm with a battery. Some people have an alarm with a AAA battery while others have an alarm with a larger battery. However, we do know that for everyone, the fear will subside. The rate in which it subsides depends on how you approach your fear cues, and one job of your clinician is to coach you in the skill of "doing nothing" to manage the situation and "relaxing with the sensations" that occur when you get anxious. That is, by not fighting an alarm reaction, that alarm reaction subsides more quickly. This is because anxiety conditions rely on feed-forward cycles. An alarm reaction is cued by a concerning situation, attention is honed to the most fearful aspects of this situation, the accompanying anxiety makes the situation feel more dangerous, and the false alarm is further cued. To short-circuit this cycle, your clinician will guide you in evaluating the actual safety of the situation and learn how not to react to symptoms with increased concern. When this happens, the alarm turns off quickly. But to achieve this, you will need some direct experiences with your feared situations. We call this experience exposure practice, and for this practice your clinician will show you ways to "lean into the fear" and practice doing nothing so that you have the chance to evaluate the situation and your competence in it more objectively.

10.7. More on Exposure Therapy

The central feature of exposure therapy is that it is an opportunity to learn from experience when you approach that experience in a mindful, systematic, and controlled way. One particular aspect of exposure therapy is discovering the difference between what one thinks (expects) will happen and what actually happens. To do this well, one has to be able to see around the many things one tells oneself about a situation and what is actually occurring in that situation. This is what we mean by the term *mindful*—an awareness of all the elements of an experience and the difference between what we say to ourselves about an experience and all the other elements of that experience. To help this process along, your clinician may ask you to specifically review your expectations about your exposure experience and then have you decide whether those things happened or not. One important feature of this process is making sure you do not decide the reality of the situation based on how you feel. Feelings are temporary, and while your therapy is dedicated to reducing anxiety, fear, and panic, during early exposure practice you will be asked to see how comfortable you can become with your false alarm while deciding if there is actual threat in the situation. To do this well, exposure needs to have a number of characteristics:

(1) The exposure is **systematic**, which means there is a specific program aimed at helping patients re-establish a sense of safety around feared cues, including careful planning as collaboration between the clinician and patient. For example, a fear of flying patient and clinician may design a list of fear cues (a picture of an airplane, being at an airport, the smell of jet fuel, a video of a flight, virtual reality exposure to a flight, taking a very short actual flight with the clinician, taking a short flight without the clinician, taking a long flight) and decide together which one to start with and on what session.
(2) The exposure is **deliberate**, which means that it is planned and initiated by the patient. Alternatively, brief exposures in the real world, such as being randomly called on to answer a question in a meeting for a patient with social anxiety, although not harmful, are not ideal to result in lasting safety learning. By planning specific exposure exercises, with a specific focus, and a specific time, the patient learns he or she control the exposure exercise rather than the exposure exercise controlling him or her.
(3) The exposure is **prolonged**, which means that you stay with it until a predetermined time has passed. Often patients may leave an exposure exercise when their fear starts to get high rather than staying in the situation and seeing that even when their fear rises, nothing catastrophic happens.
(4) The exposure is **repeated**, which is one of the most critical conditions. Facing a feared situation once is courageous but not sufficient to result in lasting change. Also, repetitions should occur close in time to work properly. For example, giving a talk once every six months is not likely to ever eliminate a fear of social rejection.

The role of your clinician is to help coach you before, during, and after exposure therapy to attend to how your exposure experiences are different from your expectations. That is, we know that individuals in exposure therapy have tried to overcome their fears on their own and were not successful. But, like almost everything, exposure therapy is different depending on how you approach it, what you pay attention to, how long you persist with it, and how you think about it later. Safety learning is active learning, and your clinician will take you through a series of learning exercises to develop a stronger and stronger sense of safety around feared cues, providing stronger and stronger tests that prove your anxiety-ridden expectations for how you will do in these situations are not accurate.

10.8. Conclusions

You have come to treatment to rid yourself of unnecessary anxiety, fear, and avoidance, and your clinician is dedicated to this goal. The process of achieving this goal involves developing a new relationship with anxiety and fear, with learning to approach these emotions as potential false alarms. Exposure therapy involves approaching your fears in a new way, learning to get more comfortable with your experience of anxiety as you develop a sense of safety in the situations with the events that have caused you distress in the past. You will be testing out your expectations, looking past your assumptions, and developing a stronger sense of resilience and confidence with both your anxiety and the situations that evoke it. This investment in safety learning (and the temporary anxiety that comes with re-entry into avoided situations) offers you the payoff of dramatically less anxiety over time and a return to full engagement in your life and your valued activities.

11
Bibliography

11.1. Overview

This chapter provides a list of key references to research papers, chapters, and books that have informed the approach to exposure therapy that we described in the previous chapters. By listing these here, we (a) underscore that our approach is rooted in theory and guided by data from studies and clinical trials that have tested the principles, efficacy, and mechanisms of action of exposure therapy and (b) acknowledge that much of our thinking about exposure therapy and its delivery has been informed by the work of our mentors, peers, and students.

11.2. Key References

Abramowitz, J. S. (1997). Effectiveness of psychological and pharmacological treatments for obsessive-compulsive disorder: A quantitative review. *Journal of Consulting and Clinical Psychology, 65*, 44–52.

Barlow, D. H. (2002). *Anxiety and its disorders: The nature and treatment of anxiety and panic* (2nd ed.). New York, NY: Guilford.

Borkovec, T. D., & Inz, J. (1990). The nature of worry in generalized anxiety disorder: A predominance of thought activity. *Behaviour Research and Therapy, 28*, 153–158.

Bouton, M. E., Westbrook, R. F., Corcoran K. A., & Maren, S. (2006). Contextual and temporal modulation of extinction: Behavioral and biological mechanisms. *Biological Psychiatry, 60*, 352–360.

Carpenter, J. K., Andrews, L. A., Witcraft, S. M., Powers, M. B., Smits, J. A., & Hofmann, S. G. (2018). Cognitive behavioral therapy for anxiety and related disorders: A meta-analysis of randomized placebo-controlled trials. *Depression and Anxiety, 35*, 502–514.

Clark, D. (1986). A cognitive approach to panic. *Behaviour Research and Therapy, 24*, 461–470.

Clark, D. M., Ehlers, A., Hackmann, A., McManus, F., Fennell, M., Grey, N., . . . Wild, J. (2006). Cognitive therapy versus exposure and applied relaxation in social phobia: A randomized controlled trial. *Journal of Consulting and Clinical Psychology, 74*, 568–578.

Craske, M. G., Kircanski, K., Zelikowsky, M., Mystkowski, J., Chowdhury, N., & Baker, A. (2008). Optimizing inhibitory learning during exposure therapy. *Behaviour Research and Therapy, 46*, 5–27.

Foa, E. B., Keane, T. M., Friedman, M. J., & Cohen, J. A. (2010). *Effective treatments for PTSD* (2nd ed.). New York, NY: Guilford.

Foa, E. B., & Kozak, M. J. (1986). Emotional processing of fear: Exposure to corrective information. *Psychological Bulletin, 99*, 20–35.

Hofmann, S. G. (2008). Cognitive processes during fear acquisition and extinction in animals and humans: Implications for exposure therapy of anxiety disorders. *Clinical Psychology Review, 28*, 199–210.

Hofmann, S. G., & Otto, M. W. (2018). *Cognitive behavioral therapy for social anxiety disorder* (2nd ed.). New York, NY: Routledge.

Kredlow, M. A., Eichenbaum, H., & Otto, M. W. (2018). Memory creation and modification: Enhancing the treatment of psychological disorders. *American Psychologist, 73*, 269–285.

Landmann, N., Kuhn, M., Piosczyk, H., Feige, B., Baglioni, C., Spiegelhalder, K., . . . Nissen, C. (2014). The reorganisation of memory during sleep. *Sleep Medicine Review, 18*, 531–541.

Margraf, J., Barlow, D. H., Clark, D.M., & Telch, M. J. (1993). Psychological treatment of panic: Work in progress on outcome, active ingredients, and follow-up. *Behaviour Research and Therapy, 31*, 1–8.

Morrison, A. S., & Heimberg, R. G. (2013). Social anxiety and social anxiety disorder. *Annual Review of Clinical Psychology, 9*, 249–274.

Myers, K. M., & Davis, M. (2007). Mechanisms of fear extinction. *Molecular Psychiatry, 12*, 120–150.

Otto, M. W., Eastman, A., Lo, S., Hearon, B. A., Bickel, W. K., Zvolensky, M., . . . Doan, S. N. (2016). Anxiety sensitivity and working memory capacity: Risk factors and targets for health behavior promotion. *Clinical Psychology Review, 49*, 67–78.

Otto, M. W., & Hofmann, S. G. (Eds.). (2010). *Avoiding treatment failures in the anxiety disorders.* New York, NY: Springer.

Otto, M. W., & Pollack, M. H. (2009). *Stopping anxiety medication* (Therapist guide, 2nd ed.). New York, NY: Oxford University Press.

Otto, M. W., Simon, N. M., Olatunji, B. O., Sung, S. C., & Pollack, M. H. (2011). *10-Minute CBT: Integrating cognitive-behavioral strategies into your practice.* New York, NY: Oxford University Press.

Otto, M. W., Smits, J. A. J., & Reese, H. E. (2005). Combined psychotherapy and pharmacotherapy for mood and anxiety disorders in adults: Review and analysis. *Clinical Psychology: Science and Practice, 12*, 72–86.

Powers, M. B., Smits, J. A. J., & Telch, M. J. (2004). Disentangling the effects of safety-behavior utilization and safety-behavior availability during exposure-based treatment: A placebo-controlled trial. *Journal of Consulting and Clinical Psychology, 72*, 448–454.

Rodebaugh, T. L., Holaway, R. M., & Heimberg, R. G. (2004). The treatment of social anxiety disorder. *Clinical Psychology Review, 24*, 883–908.

Rothbaum, B. O., & Davis, M. (2003). Applying learning principles to the treatment of post-trauma reactions. *Annals of the New York Academy of Sciences, 1008*, 112–121.

Salkovskis, P. M. (1985). Obsessional-compulsive problems: A cognitive-behavioral analysis. *Behaviour Research and Therapy, 23*, 571–583.

Sloan, T., & Telch, M. J. (2002). The effects of safety-seeking behavior and guided threat reappraisal on fear reduction during exposure: An experimental investigation. *Behaviour Research and Therapy, 40*, 235–251.

Smits, J. A., Julian, K., Rosenfield, D., & Powers, M. B. (2012). Threat reappraisal as a mediator of symptom change in cognitive-behavioral treatment of anxiety disorders: A systematic review. *Journal of Consulting and Clinical Psychology, 80*, 624–635.

Smits, J. A. J., Otto, M. W., Powers, M. B., & Baird, S. O. (Eds.). (2018). *Anxiety sensitivity: A clinical guide to assessment and treatment.* San Diego, CA: Academic Press.

Smits, J. A. J., Powers, M. B., Cho, Y., & Telch, M. T. Mechanisms of change in cognitive-behavioral treatment of panic disorder: Evidence of the fear of fear mediational hypothesis. *Journal of Consulting and Clinical Psychology, 72,* 646–652.

Smits, J. A., Zvolensky, M. J., Davis, M. L., Rosenfield, D., Marcus, B. H., Church, T. S., . . . Baird, S. O. (2016). The efficacy of vigorous-intensity exercise as an aid to smoking cessation in adults with high anxiety sensitivity: A randomized controlled trial. *Psychosomatic Medicine, 78,* 354–364.

Tolin, D. F. (2010). Is cognitive–behavioral therapy more effective than other therapies?: A meta-analytic review. *Clinical Psychology Review, 30,* 710–720.

Yamada, T, Moshier, S. J., & Otto, M. W. (2016). No site unseen: Predicting the failure to control problematic internet use among young adults. *Cognitive Behaviour Therapy, 45,* 496–500.

11.3. References for Chapter 9

Allan, N. P., Korte, K. J., Capron, D. W., Raines, A. M., & Schmidt, N. B. (2014). Factor mixture modeling of anxiety sensitivity: A three-class structure. *Psychological Assessment, 26,* 1184–1195.

Allan, N. P., Raines, A. M., Capron, D. W., Norr, A. M., Zvolensky, M. J., & Schmidt, N. B. (2014). Identification of anxiety sensitivity classes and clinical cut-scores in a sample of adult smokers: Results from a factor mixture model. *Journal of Anxiety Disorders, 28,* 696–703.

Antony, M. M., Orsillo, S. M., & Roemer, L. (2001). *Practitioners guide to empirically based measures of anxiety.* New York, NY: Kluwer Academic.

Cuming, S., Rapee, R. M., Kemp, N., Abbott, M. J., Peters, L., & Gaston, J. E. (2009). A self-report measure of subtle avoidance and safety behaviors relevant to social anxiety: Development and psychometric properties. *Journal of Anxiety Disorders, 23,* 879–883.

Donker, T., van Straten, A., Marks, I., & Cuijpers, P. (2011). Quick and easy self-rating of generalized anxiety disorder: Validity of the Dutch Web-based GAD-7, GAD-2 and GAD-SI. *Psychiatry Research, 188,* 58–64.

Feske, U., & de Beurs, E. (1997). The Panic Appraisal Inventory: Psychometric properties. *Behaviour Research and Therapy, 35,* 875–882.

Foa, E. B., Ehlers, A., Clark, D. M., Tolin, D. F., & Orsillo, S. M. (1999). The Posttraumatic Cognitions Inventory (PTCI): Development and validation. *Psychological Assessment, 11,* 303–314.

Foa, E. B., McLean, C. P., Zang, Y., Zhong, J., Powers, M. B., Kauffman, B. Y., . . . Knowles, K. (2016). Psychometric properties of the Posttraumatic Diagnostic Scale for DSM-5 (PDS-5). *Psychological Assessment, 28,* 1166–1171.

Fresco, D. M., Coles, M. E., Heimberg, R. G., Liebowitz, M. R., Hami, S., Stein, M. B., & Goetz, D. (2001). The Liebowitz Social Anxiety Scale: a comparison of the psychometric properties of self-report and clinician-administered formats. *Psychological Medicine, 31,* 1025–1035.

Kamphuis, J. H., & Telch, M. J. (1998). Assessment of strategies to manage or avoid perceived threats among panic disorder patients: The Texas Safety Maneuver Scale (TSMS). *Clinical Psychology & Psychotherapy, 5*, 177–186.

Kroenke, K., Spitzer, R. L., & Williams, J. B. W. (2001). The PHQ-9. *Journal of General Internal Medicine, 16*, 606–613.

Laposa, J. M., Collimore, K. C., Hawley, L. L., & Rector, N. A. (2015). Distress tolerance in OCD and anxiety disorders, and its relationship with anxiety sensitivity and intolerance of uncertainty. *Journal of Anxiety Disorders, 33*, 8–14.

Mitchell, M. A., Riccardi, C. J., Keough, M. E., Timpano, K. R., & Schmidt, N. B. (2013). Understanding the associations among anxiety sensitivity, distress tolerance, and discomfort intolerance: a comparison of three models. *Journal of Anxiety Disorders, 27*, 147–154.

Obsessive Compulsive Cognitions Working Group. (2005). Psychometric validation of the obsessive belief questionnaire and interpretation of intrusions inventory, Part 2: Factor analyses and testing of a brief version. *Behaviour Research and Therapy, 43*, 1527–1542.

Rassin, E., Merckelbach, H., Muris, P., & Schmidt, H. (2001). The thought–action fusion scale: Further evidence for its reliability and validity. *Behaviour Research and Therapy, 39*, 537–544.

Rosario-Campos, M. C., Miguel, E. C., Quatrano, S., Chacon, P., Ferrao, Y., Findley, D., . . . Leckman, J. F. (2006). The Dimensional Yale–Brown Obsessive-Compulsive Scale (DY-BOCS): An instrument for assessing obsessive-compulsive symptom dimensions. *Molecular Psychiatry, 11*, 495–504.

Shear, M. K., Brown, T. A., Barlow, D. H., Money, R., Sholomskas, D. E., Woods, S. W., . . . Papp, L. A. (1997). Multicenter collaborative panic disorder severity scale. *The American Journal of Psychiatry, 154*, 1571–1575.

Telch, M. J., Lucas, R. A., Smits, J. A. J., Powers, M. B., Heimberg, R., & Hart, T. (2004). Appraisal of social concerns: A cognitive assessment instrument for social phobia. *Depression and Anxiety, 19*, 217–224.

Wells, A. (1994). A multi-dimensional measure of worry: Development and preliminary validation of the anxious thoughts inventory. *Anxiety, Stress, & Coping, 6*, 289–299.

About the Authors

Dr. Jasper A. J. Smits is Professor of Psychology and Psychiatry at the University of Texas at Austin, where he directs a research lab and clinic that focus on the treatment of anxiety and related disorders. Among his core interests are developing strategies that enhance exposure therapy outcomes and the training of clinicians in the delivery of this empirically-supported intervention. Dr. Smits is a federally-funded investigator who has published over 200 articles, chapters, and books spanning his interests. He also is a member of the Scientific Council of the Anxiety and Depression Association of America, consults to industry, and provides regular workshops on the treatment of anxiety and related disorders at national and international meetings.

Dr. Mark B. Powers is Director of Trauma Research at Baylor Scott & White, conducting federally funded projects at two Level 1 Trauma Centers including Baylor University Medical Center in Dallas and Scott & White Medical Center in Temple. He collaborates with local police as a member of the Critical Incident Stress Management and Crisis/Hostage Negotiation teams. Dr. Powers is certified in prolonged exposure therapy for PTSD and Exposure with Ritual Prevention for OCD after training at the Center for the Treatment and Study of Anxiety with Dr. Edna Foa. He also served as a Beck Scholar at the Beck Institute for Cognitive Therapy and Research. He has published over 150 articles, books, and book chapters, and is Editor-in-Chief of the journal *Cognitive Behaviour Therapy*.

Dr. Michael W. Otto is Professor of Psychological and Brain Sciences and Senior Fellow at the Institute for Health System Innovation and Policy at Boston University. Dr. Otto has had a major career focus on developing and validating new psychosocial treatments for anxiety and mood disorders. His attention to principles underlying behavior-change successes includes research on addictive behaviors, medication adherence, sleep, and exercise. Across these areas of interest, Dr. Otto has published over 400 articles and 20 books. He has served as President of the Association for Behavioral and Cognitive Therapies and President of Division 12 of the American Psychological Association, and received the Division 12 award for Distinguished Scientific Contributions to Clinical Psychology.

Index

Figures are indicated by *f* following the page number.

For the benefit of digital users, indexed terms that span two pages (e.g., 52–53) may, on occasion, appear on only one of those pages.

www.ingramcontent.com/pod-product-compliance
Ingram Content Group UK Ltd.
Pitfield, Milton Keynes, MK11 3LW, UK
UKHW022019150926
475595UK00014B/308